THE LOW DOSE IMMUNOTHERAPY HANDBOOK

Recipes and Lifestyle Advice for Patients on LDA and EPD Treatment

Nicolette M. Dumke

THE LOW DOSE IMMUNOTHERAPY HANDBOOK: RECIPES AND LIFESTLYE ADVICE FOR PATIENTS ON LDA AND EPD TREATMENT

Published by
Adapt Books
Allergy Adapt, Inc.
1877 Polk Avenue
Louisville, Colorado 80027
303-666-8253

©2003 by Nicolette M. Dumke
Fourth revision – March, 2015
Printed in the United States of America

ISBN: 978-1-887624-07-7

Dedication

To Dr. W. A. Shrader, Jr.

*for his advice on the contents of
this book and for reviewing
the book for medical accuracy,*

*for his efforts to make
low dose immunotherapy
more widely available,*

*and especially for
treating his patients
with compassion.*

Disclaimer

The information contained in this book is merely intended to communicate food preparation material and information about possible treatment options which are helpful and educational to the reader. It is not intended to replace medical diagnosis or treatment, but rather to provide information and recipes which may be helpful in implementing a diet prescribed by your doctor. Please consult your physician for medical advice before embarking on any treatment or changing your diet.

The author and publisher declare that to the best of their knowledge all material in this book is accurate; however, although unknown to the author and publisher, some recipes may contain ingredients which may be harmful to some people.

There are no warranties which extend beyond the educational nature of this book, either expressed or implied, including, but not limited to, the implied warranties of merchantability, fitness for a particular purpose, or non-infringement. Therefore, the author and publisher shall have neither liability nor responsibility to any person with respect to any loss or damage alleged to be caused, directly or indirectly, by the information contained in this book.

If you do not wish to be bound by the above, you may return this book to the publisher for a full refund.

Table of Contents

The History of Low Dose Immunotherapy

In the 1960s, Dr. S. Popper in England serendipitously discovered that when he injected his patients with what he thought was the enzyme hyaluronidase in an attempt to treat their nasal polyps, their inhalant allergies disappeared. When he was unable to reproduce the same results later, he determined that it was actually a contaminant in the first batch of hyaluronidase, the enzyme beta-glucuronidase, that was responsible for the phenomenon. After his untimely death, his colleague Dr. Len McEwen developed injections of very low doses of allergens combined with beta-glucuronidase which he dubbed Enzyme Potentiated Desensitization, or EPD.

EPD was used in the United States under an Investigational Review Board in the 1990s. When the IRB expired, delays were encountered in the submission of an Investigational New Drug (IND) proposal with the FDA. As a result, the FDA banned EPD treatment in the United States in April 2001. An IND application was submitted in the fall of 2001, but bureaucratic difficulties plagued the IND trial. Therefore, an American-made injection based on the same principle as EPD was developed.

The American-made injection is compounded in a licensed American pharmacy from American-made antigens manufactured in FDA approved laboratories. The antigens used are the same as in conventional allergy desensitization shots, but in very low concentrations. These injections are called LDA for Low Dose Allergens. In addition to common allergens, LDA contains uniquely American antigens which are not present in EPD such as cottonwood, sage, mountain juniper, some New World evergreens, American perfumes, avocadoes and other "American" foods, etc. American patients have had very good results with LDA, possibly because it is custom-made for the needs of American allergy patients rather than having been developed for the allergic exposures of the British. The author of this book has had better results with LDA than EPD, perhaps due to the more complete coverage of American antigens.

How to Live with Low Dose Immunotherapy

Being a low dose immunotherapy patient can take some getting used to. Every few months it may seem like your whole life is disrupted by your treatment. However, the good health you will enjoy after a few shots makes up for the inconvenience.

Low dose immunotherapy patients participate actively in their treatment by making necessary lifestyle and dietary modifications around the time of their injections. Your doctor and his staff will instruct you about "the rules" and their individual application to you. Your doctor should also give you a copy of the *Patient Instruction Book* ("the pink book") to clarify the rules. Read this book very carefully several times, and ask your doctor or his staff any questions you have about the instructions in the book and how they apply to you. The two most helpful comments I heard from my doctor about the rules were, "The more you can do, the better off you will be," and "Be careful, but not paranoid."

Some low dose immunotherapy patients experience anxiety because they are afraid that they will, through forgetfulness or ignorance, neglect to keep one or more of the rules. Being organized, which is covered in the third chapter of this book, can help you not to forget anything and allay this anxiety. If you do accidentally break one of the rules, ask your doctor or his staff about it. Most of the time, unless a medication that adversely affects the shot is taken, these small diversions from the protocol do not cause major problems.

The application of the rules in the patient instruction book is an individual matter. For example, the book says that eczema patients may have difficulty avoiding creams and lotions and encourages them to discuss a way around this rule with their doctors. If your have eczema, your individual needs and sensitivities may change how the rules are applied for you. Your doctor also may vary how the rules apply to you with other medical conditions and in consideration of the severity of your allergies. The length of time you must avoid various substances before and after a shot may vary from person to person. The "Timetable for LDA" in recent editions of the pink book indicates this variability by using X's on the days when everyone should avoid a substance and using parentheses on the days for which you should ask your doctor if you need to avoid that substance.

Non-medical rules issues should also be discussed with your doctor. For example, when I started treatment I was concerned about having to avoid laundry detergent for a few days at shot time because my younger son was a five-year-old then and he liked to change his shirt every time he got a speck of food on it. I asked my doctor if I could use my usual brand of unscented hypoallergenic laundry products, and he said, "Yes." (Please ask your doctor which laundry detergents are acceptable for you as this can vary with your level of chemical sensitivity). Discuss any questions or concerns you have about the rules with your doctor. Both the patient instruction book and this book were written with the most sensitive patients in mind.

Low dose immunotherapy is not a quick, easy cure for your allergies and you may have ups and downs in how you feel as your treatment progresses. The patient instruction book says "Do not be discouraged if..." in more than one place, but each time I was in one of those situations, I found that I was discouraged. Reassurances from my doctor and his staff that how I was feeling was normal for the stage of treatment I was in were very helpful. Call your doctor's office if you have concerns. They may be able to help, and if what you are feeling is not normal, they should know.

Another help for discouragement is having a friend, hopefully one who is a positive person and is a few shots ahead of you in treatment, with whom to correspond or talk to on the phone. Hearing that your friend actually did survive the "downs" and went on to reach new "ups" will make you feel better mentally immediately while you patiently wait to feel better physically.

Perhaps the best way to cope with discouragement is to prepare for it in advance. When we put so much effort into our treatments, we want to get better immediately, but for many patients, it takes time to achieve good results, especially with food allergies and chemical sensitivities. Knowing this in advance will help. Also, even the best shots wear off, especially in the early stages of your treatment. When my son took his first shot at age eleven and was able to eat everything without having eczema problems two weeks after his shot, I warned him that it might not last until his next shot. Then our doctor told him the same thing. He asked me, "Why to do you guys keep telling me that?" I replied, "So if or when it happens, you won't be upset." When it happened, he was able to cope much better than some adults do.

Finally, keep your eyes on the goal of good health and the times when you will feel better. About the time my son started low dose immunotherapy treatment, we regularly listened to a radio station that played his favorite songs while riding in the car. There was one song which we heard occasionally; we turned up the volume whenever it came on because its message was meaningful to us as low dose immunotherapy patients:

"I can see clearly now; the rain is gone,
Gone are the obstacles that were in my way.
Here is the rainbow I've been waiting for,
It's gonna be a bright, bright, sunshiny day."

Look forward to and enjoy the sunshine of relief from your allergies!

Getting Organized

Trying to follow the rules in the patient instruction book can be daunting, especially when you first start treatment. If you are organized, you will find it easier to remember and follow the rules and to prepare in advance for some of the circumstances that may arise in the course of your treatments. Also, since many patients must travel to get their injections, organization helps make the trip go more smoothly.

Some patients may experience hypersensitivity or a lack of energy after their shots. If you are among this group, it is helpful to plan your schedule around the times when you may not be in top condition. Before your shot, cook and freeze the food you and your family will need the week or so after your shot. Shop ahead of time for items you will need during the period when you may be hypersensitive. Plan your work schedule to avoid exposures as much as possible. Stay home as much as possible during your hypersensitive period, and have plenty of old books, videos, correspondence, paperwork, or needlework to keep you occupied during this time.

If you travel to get your shot, preparing food to take along on the trip is very important. This is not the time to try to find a restaurant that has something you can eat after you reach your destination! Marge Jones, editor of the *Mastering Food Allergies* newsletter, cooks ground lamb and sweet potatoes and freezes them in small, one-serving-sized jars for her trip. One patient I know who stays overnight when she and her family get their shots takes along a crock pot and ingredients to make stew when they arrive at their motel. (See the crock pot stew recipe on page 22). Suggestions for other foods you may want to take on your trip are listed on page 15.

Chemically sensitive patients should plan ahead for chemical challenges such as restrooms that they may encounter while traveling. In order to avoid using scented soaps in restrooms, take wet wash cloths in plastic bags with you and use them to wash your hands after you leave the restroom. (This also will minimize the time you spend in the restroom). Be sure to provide your traveling companions with unscented soap to use in the restroom so they don't carry a perfume scent back to you on their hands after a rest stop.

If you must spend the night away from home when you get your shot, finding an acceptable place to stay can be a challenge especially if you are chemically sensitive. Ask your doctor for suggestions for where to stay. When you go to the city where you will take your shots for your initial office visit and testing, stay in one of the places your doctor suggests, and check out the other places if you are having problems where you are staying. Many motels and hotels will make special arrangements to clean your room with Bon Ami™ or baking soda and air it out before you arrive if you ask them to.

I have found it very helpful to have a "To Do List" to help me get organized and remember what I need to do before each shot. A sample of this list follows below. Many items on the list may not apply to you, and the list may not include things that you *do* need to do. This list is just given as an example for drawing up your own list which will help you to be organized, get everything done, and not worry that you have forgotten something.

SAMPLE "TO DO LIST"

4 to 6 weeks before your shot:

Order any special foods you need for your shot. (See "Sources," pages 77 to 78 and 82, for suppliers of game meat, tuber flours, etc).
Order gloves, soaps, cleaning supplies, and supplements. (See "Sources," pages 80 and 81).
Make any necessary travel arrangements or reservations.
Gather materials and supplies for reading, letter writing, needlework, etc. if you plan to stay home and do such projects after your shot. If you would like to read a new book and are chemically sensitive, ask your doctor how long before your shot it needs to out-gas.

Purchase it far enough ahead of your shot so you can air it out for the recommended time.

Check your supplies of anti-fungal medication, supplements for your shot, etc. and get any that you need.

2 weeks to 1 week before your shot:

Xerox the "Timetable for LDA" chart from the patient instruction book; add dates and any personal instructions to it.

Get a haircut if necessary.

Do baking you will need to do for your diet. Slice bread and freeze it and other baked goods.

Prepare and freeze shot-time diet foods for yourself; this is helpful in case you do not have much energy for cooking after your shot.

Make baked goods for your family (if they usually eat "homemade") so you won't have to do it when your diet is restricted.

Prepare and freeze a few meals for your family if they will not be eating the shot-time diet with you.

Prepare and freeze food for your trip if you travel to get your shot.

Hide or put "Do not use" notes on any forbidden medications or supplements (such as flax oil that you might use on vegetables without thinking) at the appropriate time before your shot. I usually write my note on tape which I use to tape the container shut.

If you do not have pets, you may do some of the cleaning tasks in the next section at this time. I always mop earlier than one week before a shot.

One week to 3 days before your shot:

Hide or put "do not use" notes on fish and flax oil at one week before your shot.

Remove pets from your house.

Mop hard surface floors using a non-toxic cleaner such as Super-Clean™. (See "Sources," page 80 for the cleaning supplies mentioned).

Clean your garbage disposal. (See "Notes and Tips," page 69).

Clean your refrigerator, dishwasher, and any other mold problem areas using a non-toxic antifungal agent such as NutriBiotic™ if your doctor allows. Clean your bathroom with SuperClean™ and/or Bon Ami™; use carbonated water on the mirrors.

Dust your house. If you feel you need to use something on your furniture, see note about furniture polishing on page 70.

Wash or vacuum rugs or carpets.

Wash or change the filters in your furnace and air cleaner.

Wash all bedding.

Vacuum your bed.

Run your pillows through the dryer.

Clean and vacuum your car.

Make tapioca wafers. (See the recipe on page 17).

If you travel to get your shot, begin packing clothes and linens.

Wash your mask if you wear one to get to your doctor's office.

Do major grocery shopping.

Get gas in your car.

Take your children (or yourself!) on an outing if you are going to stay home a lot after your shot.

2 days before your shot:

Discard or put all newspapers and magazines into plastic bags.

Hide or put a note not to use on these items:

Kitchen:

Hand soap (Replace with Magick Botanicals™ Hand and Body Wash or Simple™ Soap).

Dishwashing liquid (Replace with unscented brand, if allowed, or use Magick Botanicals™ Hand and Body Wash for washing dishes).

Dishwasher detergent

Rubber gloves (Replace with plastic gloves).

Hand lotion

Laundry room:
Laundry soaps, pre-treatments, and other laundry products (Replace with unscented products, if allowed).

Bathroom:
Water cup (Replace with a small bottle of bottled water).
Deodorant (Replace with "the rock" or baking soda).
Toothpaste (Replace with baking soda).
Soap (Replace with Magick Botanicals™ Hand and Body Wash or Simple™ Soap).
Shampoo (Replace with Magick Botanicals™ Hand and Body Wash or shampoo or Simple™ Shampoo).
Creams, lotions, and makeup

Bedroom:
Water cup on bedside table (Replace with a small bottle of water)
Computer, if less than a year old or room is poorly ventilated

The day before leaving on your trip, if you travel:

Check with the highway department for road conditions if you are traveling by car, especially in the winter.

Call the motel or hotel where you will stay and remind them of special arrangements you have made with them for cleaning and airing out your room.

Make ice for your cooler.

Finish packing clothes, pillows and/or linens.

Pack room-temperature food (tapioca wafers, bottled water, etc.)

Find all necessary food items for the trip in your freezer.

Organize refrigerated and frozen food you plan to take along so you can find it and put it in your cooler easily the next day.

Prepare stew ingredients and pack your crock pot if you plan to make crock pot stew in your motel or hotel room.

Refrigerate bottled water if you would like to take it along cold.

Get out plastic bags and wash cloths; wet the wash cloths before you leave and pack them in the bags for hand washing along the way.

Give your traveling companions non-scented soap to use in restrooms.

The day before your shot:

Bathe with Magick Botanicals™ Hand and Body Wash or Simple™
soap and shampoo.
If you are not traveling and it is possible to do so, this is a good time
to stay home and finish cooking for your diet.

After your shot:

Mark the date of your next shot on your calendar so you can schedule
around it.

SUGGESTED ITEMS TO TAKE ON YOUR TRIP
IF YOU TRAVEL TO GET YOUR SHOT

Foods:

Chilled small bottles of water and/or carbonated water
Cassava or white sweet potato bread, crackers, bagels or tortillas (See
the recipes on pages 18 to 21).
Tapioca wafers (See the recipe on page 17).
Sweet potato chips or white potato chips (See the recipe on page 35).
Cassava fries (See the recipe on page 30).
Carrot snax (See the recipe on page 34).
Jerky or meat bits (See the recipes on pages 35 and 36).
Cooked lamb, rabbit, venison, or fish
Baked sweet potatoes or white potatoes
Cooked carrots or cabbage, cold or hot (in a thermos)
Stew ingredients and a crock pot to cook them in (See the recipe on
page 22).

For patients using fructose or glycerin rather than the shot-time diet:

Hot bottled water in a thermos (to mix with the fructose or glycerin)

Chilled small bottles of water and/or carbonated water

Fructose or glycerin

Glass or cup and spoon with which to mix fructose or glycerin and water

Miscellaneous items:

Unscented soap for your traveling companions to use in restrooms

Wash cloths in Ziploc™ bags (Wet them before you leave).

Mask

Air filter for your car and/or motel or hotel room

Bedding washed with unscented soap if you are chemically sensitive and will stay overnight

Shot-Time Diet Baked Goods

The basic shot-time diet does not include any grains but it does include starchy foods that can be used as bread and cereal substitutes. One of the most important practical questions I asked as I prepared for my first shot was whether Special Foods' cassava and white sweet potato flours and baking powders would be allowed on the shot-time diet. When the answer was "Yes," I had bread! (See ordering information for Special Foods on page 82).

Foods from Special Foods are expensive, so you may wish to live on vegetables, lamb, rabbit, venison, and fish around the time of your shot. However, if you are allergic to the shot-time diet meats, foods from Special Foods and the fresh starchy tubers they are made from may give you something substantial to eat. Also, tapioca flour (also called tapioca starch or tapioca starch flour) is not expensive, so you can use the tapioca wafers, below, to add some crunch to the basic diet whatever your budget is.

Tapioca Wafers

These wafers add a starchy food to the shot-time diet for a reasonable price but can be challenging to make. They are affected by weather, humidity, variations in the flour, and the type of baking sheets used. If your wafers come out too hard to chew easily, try microwaving them for a few seconds or dunking them in boiling water or rhubarb tea.

1¼ cups tapioca flour
¼ teaspoon sea salt
½ cup plus or minus 1 tablespoon bottled water

Combine the flour and salt in a bowl. Stir in about ⅜ cup of the water. The dough is difficult to mix; you may have to stir it and then let it rest a few seconds, then stir and let it rest, etc. Add the remaining 1 to 3 tablespoons of water one tablespoon at a time until the dough is of a consistency that cracks when stirred but liquefies readily when left alone. To bake the wafers, use a dark or dull-finished baking sheet rather than a shiny one if possible, or, if your allergies allow, use a non-stick baking sheet. (Ecko "Baker's Secret™" non-stick baking sheets work the best. They are less expensive than Ecko "Pro™" baking sheets also). Sprinkle the baking sheet generously with tapioca flour or grease it with Tomor™ margarine. (This is not necessary if you use a non-stick baking sheet). Drop teaspoonfuls of the dough 2 to 3 inches apart on the baking sheet and allow the dough to spread out. If your baking sheet is not large enough to hold all of the batter, put the rest of the batter on another baking sheet immediately rather than leaving it in the bowl until the first sheet has cooked. Bake at 375ºF for 20-30 minutes, or until they begin to turn golden on the bottom. (If they stick, let them bake 2 or 3 minutes longer. If they still stick, pry them off with a spatula and/or a knife. Sticking indicates that the dough may be slightly too moist). Allow to cool for several hours or preferably overnight before packaging them. If you are not sensitive to plastic, they keep best in a Ziploc™ bag. They tend to get hard more quickly when stored in cellophane. These wafers are best eaten fairly fresh and may get hard to chew when stored for very long. Makes 1½ to 2 dozen wafers.

Shot-Time Diet Bread

The white sweet potato and cassava bread recipes which Special Foods will send you on request when you order flour may be made for the shot-time diet if you do not oil the pan. Dust the baking pan with flour *without oiling it* and then sprinkle the bottom of the pan with additional flour, or grease the pan with Tomor™ margarine before flouring it. If the bread has not pulled away from the sides of the pan at the end of the baking time given in the recipe, bake for an additional 10 minutes. Then, if needed, loosen the sides of the bread from the pan with a knife. The bread will stick less if baked in a dark metal pan rather than a shiny metal or glass baking pan.

Shot-Time Diet Crackers

White Sweet Potato:

1 cup white sweet potato flour (See "Sources," page 82).

1½ teaspoons white sweet potato baking powder (See "Sources," page 82).

¼ teaspoon sea salt

⅝ cup (½ cup plus 2 tablespoons) bottled water

Cassava:

1¼ cups cassava flour (See "Sources," page 82).

1 teaspoon cassava baking powder (See "Sources," page 82).

½ teaspoon sea salt

½ cup bottled water

Choose one set of ingredients, above. Combine the flour, baking powder, and salt in a bowl. Stir in the water until it is completely mixed in. Sprinkle a little flour on a baking sheet. Put the dough on the baking sheet, sprinkle the top of it with more flour, and pat and/or roll it out to about ⅛ inch thickness, dusting the top of the dough with more flour as needed while you are rolling it out. Cut into 1½ inch squares. Sprinkle with additional salt if desired. Bake at 350°F for 10 to 14 minutes for white sweet potato crackers or for 14 to 18 minutes for cassava crackers. Remove the crackers from the baking sheet with a spatula and cool them on a wire rack. Makes about 3 dozen crackers.

Shot-Time Diet Tortillas

White Sweet Potato:

1 cup white sweet potato flour (See "Sources," page 82).

¼ teaspoon sea salt

½ cup bottled water

Cassava:

1¼ cups cassava flour (See "Sources," page 82).
⅜ teaspoon sea salt
½ cup bottled water

Choose one set of ingredients, above. Stir together the flour and salt. Add the water and stir and knead to form a dough about the consistency of Play-doh™. Divide the dough into 8 portions. Roll each portion into a ball, flour it well, and put it between two sheets of cellophane (or parchment paper, plastic wrap or waxed paper if you are not sensitive to them). Roll it out with a rolling pin to about 1/16 to ⅛ inch thickness. Heat a heavy frying pan over medium heat. (Add no oil). One at a time, put each tortilla into the pan and cook it until the top is dry and it begins to brown in spots on the underside. Turn it with a spatula and cook it until the second side begins to brown also. (If you are not sensitive to coatings such as Teflon, an electric tortilla maker is an easy and quick way to make these tortillas. See "Sources," page 82). After cooking, cool the tortillas on a dishtowel or wire rack. Makes 8 tortillas. Serve plain or as "Burritos," page 23.

Shot-Time Diet Bagels

White Sweet Potato/Tapioca:

1 cup white sweet potato flour (See "Sources," page 82).
½ cup tapioca flour
2 teaspoons white sweet potato baking powder (See "Sources," page 82).
¼ teaspoon sea salt plus additional sea salt for cooking water
⅔ cup bottled water plus additional bottled water for cooking
Tomor™ margarine - about 2 teaspoons (See the margarine note on page 68. Not needed if you use a non-stick baking sheet).

Cassava:

1½ cups cassava flour (See "Sources," page 82).
2¼ teaspoons cassava baking powder (See "Sources," page 82).
¼ teaspoon sea salt plus additional sea salt for cooking water
¾ cup bottled water plus additional bottled water for cooking
Tomor™ margarine - about 2 teaspoons (See the note about this
margarine on page 68. Not needed if you use a non-stick
baking sheet).

Choose one set of ingredients, above. Put bottled water into a large saucepan to a depth of at least 2 inches. Add ¼ teaspoon sea salt per quart of water. Bring the water to a boil; then turn off the heat. Grease a baking sheet with margarine or use a non-stick baking sheet. Turn on your broiler to 500°F.

Stir together the flour(s), baking powder, and ¼ teaspoon salt. Stir in the measured amount of water listed in the ingredients until just mixed. Working quickly, divide the dough into fourths. Pick up each piece in your hands, form it into a ball, and make a hole in the center with your finger. Put each bagel on the prepared baking sheet. Broil the bagels about 5 inches from the heat for 3 minutes. CAREFULLY turn them with a spatula and broil the other side for three minutes. When you start broiling the bagels, turn on the heat under the water again. When it comes to a boil, reduce the heat to a simmer. After broiling them, carefully transfer the bagels to the boiling water and put the lid on the pan. Simmer the cassava bagels for four minutes or the sweet potato bagels for two minutes. Preheat your oven to 350°F while the bagels are boiling. Remove the bagels from the water with a slotted spatula and put them back on the baking sheet. Bake the cassava bagels for 1 hour and 10 minutes and the sweet potato bagels for 1 hour. Remove the bagels to a wire rack and cool thoroughly before slicing. Makes 4 bagels.

Main and Side Dishes for the Shot-Time Diet

There are several main and side dish recipes for the shot-time diet in the back of the patient instruction book, but it is nice to have more variety when the number of foods on your diet is limited. Lamb, venison, fish, rabbit, and vegetables don't have to be boring!

Crock Pot Shot-Time Diet Stew

2 pounds of lamb or venison cut into 1 inch cubes
5 carrots (about 1 pound) peeled and cut into 1 inch pieces
5 stalks of celery cut into 1 inch pieces
3 to 4 potatoes peeled and cut into cubes (about 1½ pounds, optional)
½ cup granulated tapioca
2 teaspoons sea salt
2¼ cups bottled water

If time permits and you would like to have a rich-colored stew, rub a skillet with a fat edge of the meat and brown the meat cubes in the skillet using no oil. (Browning the meat is not necessary if you are short on time or are making this stew in a hotel room while traveling to get your shot). Combine the meat with the vegetables, tapioca, salt, and water in a 3-quart crock pot. Stir the mixture well to evenly distribute the tapioca. Cook it on low for 8 to 10 hours or on high for 6 hours, adding more water near the end of the cooking time if you prefer a juicier stew. This stew freezes well. Makes 6 to 8 servings.

Parsnip Stew Variation: Substitute 2 pounds parsnips (about 6 cups of 1 inch pieces) for the vegetables above. Increase the water to 3 cups.

Stroganoff

1 pound lamb or venison cut into ½ inch by 1½ inch strips OR
     1 pound ground lamb or venison
1¼ cups bottled water, divided
¼ teaspoon sea salt, or to taste
1 tablespoon tapioca flour
Cooked white sweet potato or cassava noodles (See "Sources," page
     82) or mashed potatoes, white sweet potatoes, or cassava
     roots (recipe on page 29)

If you are using the meat strips, rub a fat edge of the meat around the inside of a skillet. Cook the meat strips or ground meat over medium heat, stirring occasionally, until brown. Drain almost all of the fat. Stir in the salt and 1 cup of the water and simmer for 5 to 10 minutes. Stir together the remaining ¼ cup water and the tapioca flour and add them to the skillet. Cook until the mixture returns to a boil and thickens. Serve over cooked noodles or mashed vegetables. Makes 4 to 6 servings.

Burritos

1 batch of cassava or white sweet potato tortillas, page 19
¾ pound ground lamb or venison OR cooked lamb, venison,
     or fish
1 to 2 cup cooked shot-time diet vegetables (optional)

Make the tortillas as directed in the recipe. While cooking them, brown the uncooked ground meat in a skillet, salting to taste if desired. Add the vegetables and warm through. If you are using cooked meat or fish, combine it with the vegetables and a very small amount of bottled water in a pan and warm them until the water evaporates. Place some of the meat mixture down the center of each tortilla and fold both sides over the meat. Makes 8 burritos.

Fish Cakes

1 pound of any fresh fish cut into chunks
¼ teaspoon sea salt (optional)
2 tablespoons bottled water
½ cup tapioca flour, divided

Combine the fish and water in a food processor and process until blended. Sprinkle ¼ to ⅓ cup of the tapioca flour (enough so the mixture is not real wet) over the fish and process again about a minute, until well blended. Turn out onto a plate sprinkled with tapioca flour, and shape into four patties about ¾ inch thick. Preheat a non-stick skillet. "Dry fry" patties quickly over medium heat, cooking until both sides are light brown, for 10 minutes total cooking time. Makes 4 servings.

Easy Poached Fish

Fish fillet(s) or steak(s)
Bottled water
Sea salt

Place the fish in a single layer in a casserole dish with a lid. Add bottled water to a depth of ½ inch and salt to taste. Bake at 350°F for 15 to 25 minutes (longer for thicker fish), or until the fish flakes easily.

Lamb or Venison Nuggets

1 pound ground lamb or venison
½ teaspoon sea salt
Tapioca flour – about ¼ cup

Mix the salt into the meat and divide the meat into 12 portions. Roll each part into a ball and flatten it to about ½ inch thickness.

Coat the entire outside surface with tapioca flour. Put the nuggets in a skillet and cook them over medium heat for 5 to 10 minutes, or until they are brown on the first side. Turn and cook an additional 5 to 10 minutes or until the second side is brown. Serve plain or with rhubarb jam, page 37, as a sauce for dipping. Makes 4 servings.

Tender Ground Venison

This is delicious served over mashed potatoes (page 29) or baked potatoes which have been cut in half and mashed with a fork.

1 pound ground venison
¾ to 1 teaspoon sea salt
Bottled water

Brown the meat in a skillet over medium heat, stirring frequently and breaking it up into small pieces as it cooks. When the pink color is gone, add the salt and enough water to nearly come to the top of the meat in the pan. Cover the skillet with its lid and bring it to a boil. Reduce the heat and simmer it for 30 to 45 minutes, stirring occasionally, until the water is completely evaporated. This cooking method thoroughly tenderizes the venison, which may make it acceptable to children who have an aversion to meat that is difficult for them to chew.

Skillet Hash

1 pound ground lamb or venison
3 cups chopped potatoes, boiled or baked and peeled
¾ teaspoon salt, or to taste
¼ to ½ cup bottled water

Brown the meat in a skillet over medium heat, stirring frequently. Drain all but about 2 tablespoons of the fat. Stir in the potatoes and salt. Cook over medium heat for 10 to 15 minutes, turning with a spatula as the bottom browns. Add the water to the pan. When the water begins to steam, reduce the heat to low, cover the pan, and cook the hash for another 10 minutes or until the water is gone. Makes 4 to 6 servings.

Braised Venison Burgers

If you try to broil venison "well done," it will probably be tough. Steaks are safe to eat rare, but for burgers, use this recipe.

1 pound ground venison
½ teaspoon sea salt
Bottled water

Mix the meat and salt together with your hands; form into 4 patties. Place them in a glass baking dish with a cover and add water to a depth of ½ inch. Cover with the lid and bake at 350°F for 45 minutes. Uncover and bake for 15 minutes, or until the tops of the burgers begin to brown. Turn the burgers with a spatula and bake for an additional 15 minutes, or until the second side begins to brown. Makes 4 servings.

Braised Rabbit

1 rabbit (about 3 pounds)
¼ to ½ teaspoon sea salt, or to taste
¾ cup bottled water

Cut the rabbit into serving-sized pieces, and put them in a 9 by 13 inch baking dish. Pour the water into the bottom of the dish and sprinkle the rabbit with the salt. Cover the dish with its lid or with foil and bake at 350°F for 1 hour. Uncover and bake and additional ½ to 1 hour, or until the rabbit is brown and the liquid has evaporated. Makes 4 to 6 servings.

Slow Roasted Rabbit

1 rabbit (about 3 pounds)
1 tablespoon bottled water
¼ to ½ teaspoon sea salt, or to taste

Cut the rabbit into serving-sized pieces. Put the water in the bottom of a 3-quart crock pot. Add the rabbit pieces and sprinkle them with the salt. Cover and cook on high for 1 hour, then reduce the heat to low and cook for another 7 to 10 hours. If you are at home, you may want to move the pieces on the top in the pot to the bottom and the pieces on the bottom to the top halfway through the cooking time so all of the pieces brown. Do not open the pot to check the rabbit often, though. Reserve the broth in the pot at the end of the cooking time for "Quick Rabbit Soup," page 28. Makes 4 to 6 servings.

Quick Rabbit Soup

About 1 cup broth reserved from "Slow Roasted Rabbit," page 27
¼ to ½ cup cooked carrots, celery, parsnips, cabbage, or a mixture
    of these vegetables cut into small pieces
¼ to ⅓ cup diced cooked rabbit

Combine all ingredients in a saucepan and heat to boiling. Makes one serving.

Celery Soup

1 large bunch of celery, about 1½ pounds
4 cups bottled water
1½ teaspoons sea salt

Clean the celery and slice it into ¼ inch to ½ inch slices. Place it in a saucepan with the water and salt, bring to a boil, and simmer 10 to 15 minutes. Remove about 1 cup of the celery. Puree the remaining celery and water. Return the reserved celery to the pan with the puree. Heat and serve. Makes about 1½ quarts of soup or 4 servings.

Vegetable Soup

2 to 2¼ pounds red potatoes
½ to ⅝ pound celery with leaves
½ pound carrots
6 cups bottled water
1¾ to 2¼ teaspoons sea salt or to taste.

Peel the potatoes and trim off any bad spots. Cut them into cubes. Combine them with water and salt in a saucepan and bring to a boil. Reduce the heat and simmer them for about 5 minutes while you are preparing the carrots and celery.

Peel the carrots and trim the celery. Slice them. Cut the celery leaves into small pieces. Add the prepared vegetables to the pan with the potatoes and return it to a boil. Reduce the heat and simmer for about 20 minutes or until the vegetables are tender. Makes 5 to 6 servings.

Carrot-Parsnip Medley

3 cups shredded carrots (3 large, about ¾ pound)
3 cups shredded parsnips (3 large, about ¾ pound)
¾ cup water
¼ teaspoon sea salt, or to taste

Combine all of the ingredients in a covered saucepan. Bring them to a boil, reduce the heat to medium, and cook for 10 minutes, stirring occasionally. Makes 6 servings.

Mashed White or Sweet Potatoes or Cassava Roots

6 medium sized white potatoes, 4 medium sweet potatoes, or 2 to 3 cassava roots*, or about 2 pounds of potatoes or roots

4 cups water

1 to 1½ teaspoons sea salt, divided, or to taste

3 tablespoons of Tomor™ margarine (optional, or substitute a tolerated oil if you are using this for "eating exotic" or the VMD)

⅓ to ½ cup water for the white or sweet potatoes or 1 to 1½ cups water for the mashed cassava roots.

Wash and peel or scrub the white or sweet potatoes. Peel the cassava roots. Cut the potatoes or roots into smaller cubes which will cook quickly. Put them in a saucepan with the 4 cups of water and ½ teaspoon of the salt and cover the pan. Bring them to a boil over medium heat. Reduce the heat and simmer them for 20 to 45 minutes, or until they are tender when pierced with a fork. Pour off the water and reserve it, measure out the amount of water needed for the type of potatoes you are cooking. Add the reserved water, optional margarine (or oil if you are not making these for the 3-day diet), and ½ teaspoon of salt to the pan and mash with a potato masher. Taste them and add the remaining ½ teaspoon salt if needed. If they seem dry, add more water and mash it in. Makes 4 to 6 servings.

NOTE on cassava: Fresh cassava roots can be purchased at international markets and some Safeway stores. See "Sources," page 77, for the phone number of a producer of cassava which may be able to tell you where to purchase them in your area.

Cassava Fries

1 cassava (yucca) root, about 1 pound (See "Sources, page 77).
¼ teaspoon sea salt
1 tablespoon melted Tomor™ margarine (optional – see note)

Wash the cassava root and pierce it in several places with a knife. Put it on a piece of aluminum foil on a baking sheet and bake at 350°F for 30 minutes. Remove the root from the oven and dry it with paper towels to remove as much as possible of the waxy coating that it may have come with. Discard the aluminum foil which may contain melted wax. Allow the root to cool until it is easy to handle. Peel it and cut it into ⅜ to ½ inch sticks or fries. Cassava roots may have a fibrous string down the middle of the root; if you are making these fries for children or fussy eaters, you may wish to remove this string while you are cutting the root into fries. Toss the sticks with the salt and optional margarine or oil and spread them in a single layer on a baking sheet (preferably non-stick if you are not using the oil or margarine). Bake at 400°F for 30 to 40 minutes, turning them over halfway through the baking time, until light brown on both the top and bottom sides. Do not over-bake these fries or they may be very hard rather than tender in the center. Makes 3 to 4 servings.

NOTE on using Tomor™ margarine in this recipe and the next recipe: If you are making these fries to "eat exotic" or have on your very mixed diet, substitute a tolerated oil. For the EPD or LDA critical time diet, the only fat allowed is Tomor™ or Granose™ margarine.

White or Sweet Potato Fries

4 medium-sized white potatoes or sweet potatoes*, about 2 pounds
½ teaspoon sea salt
2 tablespoons melted Tomor™ margarine (optional - see note above)

Peel the potatoes and cut them into ⅜ to ½ inch sticks or fries. (If you wish to do this ahead of time, cover them with cold water and refrigerate; then dry them with towels). Toss the potato sticks with the salt and margarine and spread them in a single layer on a baking sheet (preferably non-stick if you are not using the margarine). Bake at 400°F for 30 to 40 minutes, turning occasionally, until brown on all sides. Makes 4 to 6 servings.

NOTE on sweet potatoes – These fries are best made with white sweet potatoes, also called Jersey sweet potatoes, which are more mealy and less sweet than orange sweet potatoes. Orange sweet potatoes may be called "yams" although they are not true yams.

Shot-Time Diet Hot Cereal or Side Dish

⅓ cup cream of white sweet potato or cream of cassava cereal
    (See "Sources," page 82).
1¼ cups bottled water
Dash of sea salt

Moisten the cereal with ½ cup of the water. Put the remaining ¾ cup of the water and the salt in a saucepan and bring them to a boil. Stir in the cereal, return to a boil, lower the heat, and simmer for 5 minutes. Remove from the heat and allow to stand for an additional 5 minutes before serving (if you can wait). Makes one serving as a breakfast cereal or two as a side dish.

Creamy Cereal Variation: Substitute ⅓ cup white sweet potato or cassava flour for the cereal called for in the recipe and prepare as directed above.

Tapioca Hot Cereal or Side Dish

½ cup small pearl tapioca
2 cups bottled water
Sea salt to taste

Combine the tapioca and water in a saucepan and allow to stand overnight. In the morning, bring to a boil and simmer for 10 to 15 minutes, or until most of the tapioca pearls are clear. Add salt to taste. Makes 3 to 5 servings.

Cassava Meal Mush

1⅓ cups cassava meal (See "Sources," page 77).
4 cups bottled water
1 teaspoon sea salt, or to taste

Stir together the cassava meal with 2 cups of cold water in a small bowl. Put the remaining 2 cups of water and the salt in a large saucepan and bring it to a boil. Add the wet cassava meal to the boiling water a little at a time, stirring the mush constantly. Return to a boil; then reduce the heat to a low simmer and cook it over very low heat for 30 minutes. Stir the mush thoroughly every five minutes while it is cooking. It will be very stiff when it is done. Makes 4 to 6 servings.

Tossed Salad

2 cups lettuce, torn into bite-sized pieces
⅛ to ¼ cup cooked carrots, cut into small pieces (optional)
Dash sea salt
1 teaspoon rhubarb concentrate, page 36, or more to taste

In a serving bowl, sprinkle the lettuce and carrots with the sea salt and rhubarb concentrate. Toss thoroughly. Makes 1 serving.

Desserts, Snacks, and Beverages for the Shot-Time Diet

One of the hardest things about the shot-time diet, especially for children, is that it doesn't contain many treats or snacks. When my son was young, he liked to snack on tapioca wafers, page 16, and the recipes in this chapter.

Rhubarb Pudding

1 pound rhubarb (about 4 cups ½-inch slices)
1¼ cups bottled water, divided
3 tablespoons granulated tapioca

Clean the rhubarb and cut it into ½ inch slices. Place it in a saucepan with ¾ cup of the water. Bring it to a boil, reduce the heat, and simmer, covered, for 10 to 15 minutes, or until the rhubarb is tender. While it is simmering, combine the tapioca with the remaining ½ cup water and allow them to stand for at least 5 minutes. Then add the tapioca mixture to the rhubarb, return it to a boil, and simmer for 5 minutes. Cool the pudding for at least 20 minutes before serving. It will thicken as it cools. Makes 4 to 6 servings.

NOTE: For the third or fourth and following days after your shot or for "eating exotic," you may wish to add white stevia powder, ⅛ teaspoon or to taste, to the pudding to sweeten it when you add the tapioca mixture. (See "Sources," page 81).

Parsnip-Rhubarb Pudding

½ pound parsnips, or about 2¼ cups 1-inch pieces
¼ pound rhubarb, or about 1¼ cups 1-inch pieces
2¾ cups bottled water, divided
3 tablespoons granulated tapioca

Peel the parsnips. Cut the rhubarb and parsnips into 1 inch pieces. Combine them with 2¼ cups of the water in a saucepan, bring to a boil, and cook over medium hear until soft, about 25 minutes. While they are cooking, soak the tapioca in the remaining ½ cup water for at least 5 minutes. Allow the vegetables to cool slightly and puree them with a hand blender, blender, or food processor. Combine them with the tapioca mixture in the saucepan, return the mixture to a boil, and simmer for 5 minutes. Cool the pudding for at least 20 minutes before serving. Makes 4 to 6 servings.

Parsnip-Rhubarb "Ice Cream"

Make parsnip-rhubarb pudding above, and freeze all but ½ cup of it in ice cube trays for several hours or overnight. Refrigerate the reserved ½ cup of pudding. Remove the ice cube trays from the freezer and allow them to stand at room temperature for about ½ hour, or until the cubes soften slightly. Put the reserved pudding into a food processor or blender. Add the frozen cubes one at a time, processing after each addition, until all the cubes are added and the "ice cream" is smooth. Makes 2½ to 3 cups or 4 to 6 servings of creamy frozen dessert which is surprisingly good.

Carrot Snax

Large-diameter carrots
Bottled water

Peel the carrots and slice them about ¼ inch thick. Put them in a saucepan with water to cover. Bring to a boil, reduce the heat, and simmer for 10 to 12 minutes, or until crisp-tender. Drain the carrots and place the slices on dehydrator trays. Dry them in a dehydrator at 125°F (or whatever temperature is specified in your dehydrator instruction book) for 7 to 10 hours or until leathery. One pound of carrots yields about 1 ounce of carrot snax. If you are pressed for time, you may use frozen sliced carrots instead of fresh carrots, although they are easier to over-dry and of lower quality .

To oven dry: Cover your oven rack(s) with four thicknesses of nylon net and securely pin the edges of the net over the edges of the racks. Preheat your oven to 175°F. After boiling the carrot slices, place them on the net and put the rack(s) in the oven as far from the heating elements that are operating as possible. (In my oven, only the bottom element comes on when it is set on "bake," so I use the highest position for the racks). Put a thermometer near the back of the rack you are using and prop the oven door open about 4 inches. Set the oven to whatever temperature will maintain a temperature of 120°F to 140°F on the thermometer. (This is between 160°F and 175°F for my oven). Do not leave the drying process unattended. Check the oven temperature and progress of the carrots frequently, reducing the temperature setting to maintain the right thermometer reading as the drying progresses. It will take about 14 hours to dry carrots this way.

Sweet or White Potato Chips

Peel and thinly slice orange or white sweet potatoes or white potatoes. Place the slices on a wire rack with a baking sheet underneath it and sprinkle them with sea salt. Bake at 350°F for 30 minutes. Then broil them at 400°F about 5 inches from the heating element for 2 to 3 minutes on each side, or until they lightly brown.

Meat Bits

Lean lamb (such as leg) or venison
Sea salt, about 1 teaspoon per pound of meat

Trim the fat off of the meat and cut it into ½ inch cubes with an electric knife. Rub a baking sheet with some of the fat. Spread the meat cubes on the sheet in a single layer and sprinkle them with sea salt. Bake at 200°F, turning occasionally with a spatula, until they are dry and chewy, about 2½ to 3½ hours. Store in the refrigerator or freezer. Each pound of meat makes about 6 ounces of meat bits.

Jerky

Lean lamb (such as leg), venison, or fish (good made with salmon)
Sea salt, about 1 teaspoon per pound of meat or fish

Remove the bones and fat from the meat or the skin and bones from the fish and freeze overnight. Remove from the freezer and allow to thaw partially. Slice ¼ inch thick with an electric knife. (For the meat, if you slice with the grain, your jerky will be more leathery; if you slice against the grain, it will break more easily and be easier to chew). Sprinkle both sides of the slices with the salt. Layer them in a bowl, cover, and refrigerate several hours or overnight. Place the meat or fish on dehydrator trays and dehydrate at 145°F (or whatever temperature is specified in your dehydrator instruction book) for 12 to 14 hours or until the jerky is leathery. While drying, occasionally blot with paper towel to remove beads of oil. When the jerky is dry, there should be no moist spots. For meat cut with the grain, when the jerky is bent, it should crack but not break. Use within several days or store in the refrigerator or freezer. One pound of meat or fish yields 3 to 4 ounces of jerky.

Oven drying is not recommended for jerky. If you do not have a dehydrator, make "Meat Bits," page 35, instead of jerky.

Rhubarb Concentrate

1 pound rhubarb
2 cups bottled water

Clean the rhubarb and cut it into ½ inch slices. Place it in a saucepan with the water. Bring it to a boil, reduce the heat, and simmer, covered, for one hour. Pour the mixture into a strainer or colander and let it stand for about ½ hour to thoroughly strain the liquid from the rhubarb slices. Reserve the slices to use in "Rhubarb Jam" on the next page. Use rhubarb concentrate to make rhubarb tea on the next page or as the acid component in leavening for baking. (See "Notes," page 67, for how to use it as leavening during the three weeks after a shot when the amount of vitamin C must be limited). Refrigerate concentrate to use within a few days or freeze any leftover rhubarb concentrate for future use.

Rhubarb Tea

Rhubarb concentrate, page 36
Bottled water, boiling

Put 4 to 6 tablespoons of rhubarb concentrate into a 10-ounce mug and fill with boiling water to make rhubarb tea. One batch of rhubarb concentrate makes about 6 to 8 cups of a tangy tea somewhat like rosehip or hibiscus tea.

Rhubarb Jam

Prepare and cook rhubarb as for rhubarb concentrate, page 36. After straining off the liquid, puree the reserved rhubarb slices with a food processor or blender until smooth. Serve on tapioca wafers, white sweet potato or cassava crackers, tortillas, or bread, pages 17 to 21, or use as a dipping sauce for lamb nuggets, page 24. Makes 1 cup of jam.

NOTE: For the third to fourth and following days after your shot, you may add ⅛ teaspoon stevia powder or more to taste to each cup of rhubarb jam to sweeten it. (See "Sources," page 81.)

Recipes for Eating Exotic

Eating exotic is a solution to two problems that may occur in the course of low dose immunotherapy treatment. Some patients are allergic to almost all foods but are able to eat fairly normally as long as they take neutralization treatment. Others must follow a very strict rotation diet and will react to their "safe" foods when they upset the careful "masking balance" of the diet around the time of their shots. When these patients have to give up their neutralizing drops or shots before starting their treatment or disrupt the balance of their rotation diets, exotic or rare foods which they have not previously eaten may give them something to eat that will not cause symptoms.

Also, a few patients experience a hypersensitive period with foods for up to three weeks, or rarely longer, after their shots. After my first shot, I found that some foods that I had considered safe and had used as staples of my diet, such as amaranth, quinoa, and sweet potatoes, were causing symptoms. After the nurse at my doctor's office reassured me that this was a normal thing to have happen, I began eating exotic to get through my hypersensitive period and still feel all right. A different take on eating exotic that your doctor may recommend is to eat small amounts of many exotic foods, rotating them if possible, as a very mixed or "crazy rotation" diet. (See page 45 for more about this).

For exotic grain substitutes, you may want to try Special Foods' flours. Although expensive, malanga, true yam, lotus, water chestnut, etc. provide starchy foods that you will probably tolerate because you have rarely, if ever, eaten them before. Recipes using Special Foods' cassava and white sweet potato flour are found on pages 18 to 21 of this book. Additional recipes using other Special Foods' products follow in this chapter and on pages 47 to 49. Special Foods offers more recipes free of charge if requested when you order.

Some patients may not need to eat foods as exotic as Special Foods' products during their hypersensitive period. The more common, less expensive non-grains, such as amaranth, quinoa, and chestnut flour may be tolerated. For sources of these foods and recipes using them, refer to *The Ultimate Food Allergy Cookbook and Survival Guide*. Gluten-free grains may also be an option. For non-gluten grain recipes, refer to *The Ultimate Food Allergy Cookbook and Survival Guide*. For more about the book and how to order it, see the last few pages of this book.

For exotic protein foods, you may wish to try elk, llama, alpaca, kangaroo, antelope, goat, buffalo, duck, rabbit, alligator, rattlesnake, or types of fish that you have rarely eaten. (See "Sources," page 78). A few recipes follow; recipes for the foods not here can be found in *The Ultimate Food Allergy Cookbook and Survival Guide*.

If you eat fish, be sure to purchase it fresh from a health food store committed to organic foods because sometimes fish is treated with chemicals to extend its "freshness." Especially in inland areas, fish that was frozen immediately after it was caught may be a chemically safer choice. Fish may be broiled, with or without oil, or poached as on page 27.

Many supermarkets carry vegetables that we rarely eat such as jicama, plantain, artichokes, fennel, cassava root, etc. For instructions on how to purchase and prepare both common and unusual vegetables, refer to *The Yeast Connection Cookbook* or *Easy Cooking for Special Diets*. For more about *Easy Cooking for Special Diets*, see the last few pages of this book.

Many patients avoid fruit around the time of their shots because of *Candida* problems. However, if you can eat fruit at this time, you may want to try some of the unusual types found in many supermarkets, such as carambola, Asian pear, papaya, mango, and kiwi. If you want an easy exotic dessert, make the stevia-sweetened kiwi sorbet recipe in *The Ultimate Food Allergy Cookbook and Survival Guide*.

Exotic Hot Cereal or Side Dish

¼ cup cream of yam or ⅓ cup cream of white sweet potato, malanga, or cassava cereal from Special Foods (See "Sources," page 82).
1¼ cups water
Dash of sea salt

Moisten the cereal with ½ cup of the water. Put the remaining ¾ cup of the water and the salt in a saucepan and bring them to a boil. Stir in the cereal, return to a boil, lower the heat, and simmer for 5 minutes. Remove from the heat and allow to stand for an additional 5 minutes before serving (if you can wait). Serve with oil if desired. Makes one serving as a breakfast cereal or two as a side dish.

Special Foods' Pasta

2 cups cassava, malanga, white sweet potato, true yam, or other
    Special Foods' pasta (See "Sources," page 82).
Bottled water with a dash of sea salt
1 tablespoon oil (optional)

Fill a 3-quart saucepan about ¾ full with bottled water, add the salt, and bring to a boil. Add the pasta and return to a boil. Reduce the heat and simmer five minutes for spaghetti or noodles. (Macaroni takes slightly longer). Drain in a colander, put the pasta into a serving bowl, and toss with the oil. Serve topped with cooked exotic meat or vegetables if desired. Makes one or two servings.

Nut or Seed Waffles

1 cup walnuts, filberts, cashews, blanched almonds or other nuts*
    or sunflower seeds, sesame seeds, or pumpkin seeds
1¾ cups arrowroot, tapioca, or water chestnut flour (See
    "Sources," page 82, for water chestnut flour).
⅛ teaspoon sea salt
1¾ cups bottled water
1 tablespoon oil (optional)

Put the nuts or seeds and ½ cup of the arrowroot, water chestnut, or tapioca flour in a food processor and process until the nuts are finely ground. (You can also do this in a blender in small batches). Add the rest of the arrowroot, water chestnut, or tapioca flour and salt and process for a few seconds. With the processor running, add the water and oil and process briefly. The batter will be thin. Let the batter stand for 15 minutes while heating your waffle iron to "high." Process the batter for a few seconds each time before removing batter to cook in the iron. Use about 1½ cups batter for a 9 inch square waffle. Bake each waffle for about 15 minutes. Makes two 9 inch square 4-sectioned waffles.

NOTE: Nuts should not be used the week after your shot if you are sensitive to tree pollen; use seeds instead.

Crunchy Cassava Meal Crackers

2 cups cassava meal (See "Sources," page 77).
½ teaspoon baking soda
½ teaspoon cream of tartar
¼ teaspoon salt
¾ cup water
¼ cup oil

Preheat your over to 375°F. Oil a 12-inch by 15-inch pan. In a large bowl, mix together the cassava meal, baking soda, cream of tartar, and salt. Stir the oil into the water in a separate bowl or cup. Pour the liquid ingredients into the dry mixture and stir thoroughly. Press the crumbly mixture firmly into a 12-inch by 15-inch pan. The crumb layer will be between ⅛ and ¼ inch thick. "Cut" the crumbs into 1½ inch squares using a sharp knife. Bake the crackers for 35 to 40 minutes or until they are beginning to brown. Remove them from the pan with a spatula and put them on paper towels to cool. Makes about 3 dozen crackers.

Braised Exotic Burgers

1 pound ground buffalo or other game meat
½ teaspoon sea salt
Bottled water

Mix the meat and salt together with your hands; form into 4 patties. Place them in a glass baking dish with a cover and add water to a depth of ½ inch. Cover with the lid and bake at 350°F for 45 minutes. Uncover and bake for 15 minutes, or until the tops of the burgers begin to brown. Turn the burgers with a spatula and bake for an additional 15 minutes, or until the second side begins to brown. Makes 4 servings.

Braised Exotic Steak

Buffalo or other game meat steak
Bottled water
⅛ to ¼ teaspoon sea salt per steak, or to taste

Put the steak into a glass baking dish with a cover. Add water to a depth of ¼ inch and sprinkle with salt. Cover with the lid and bake at 350°F for 1 to 1½ hours, or until the meat is tender. If you wish to have it brown on both sides, uncover and bake an additional 20 minutes or until the water is gone.

Artichokes

Artichoke(s)
Bottled water

Trim off the stem of the artichoke(s), any bad leaves, and the tiny leaves at the bottom. (Although often recommended, it is not really necessary to cut off the spiny tips of the leaves if you eat your artichokes carefully). Place the artichokes in a saucepan with water to cover. Bring to a boil, reduce the heat, and simmer for 30 to 40 minutes, or until the stem end is tender when pierced with a fork. To eat, peel off the leaves and dip the edible end in one of the dips below if desired. Pull off the edible part between your teeth.

Oil Dip for Artichokes

For each serving, mix 2 tablespoons oil with a dash of sea salt and pepper (if tolerated).

Creamy Dip for Artichokes

¼ cup cashew, almond, or macadamia nut butter
¼ cup rhubarb concentrate, page 36, or lemon or lime juice,
    if tolerated
⅛ teaspoon salt
¼ cup oil

Puree the nut butter and rhubarb concentrate or lemon or lime juice in a blender or food processor. Add the salt and blend. With the machine running, pour in the oil in a slow stream. Makes about ¾ cup dip, or enough for about four artichokes. Do not eat this nut-containing dip within one week after your shot if you are allergic to trees.

Additional vegetable ideas:

Try these recipes in *The Ultimate Food Allergy Cookbook and Survival Guide*. (See the last pages of this book to order).

Cooked Plantains, page 110
Braised Fennel, page 113
Exotic Tubers, page 112
    These are made with cassava (yucca) root and taro root. If you live in an area with an international market, shop there for these vegetables and also true yam.

About the Very Mixed Diet

There are two situations in which the very mixed diet (VMD) – a formal system of eating a little bit of a lot of foods at each meal – can be helpful to low dose immunotherapy patients. The first is when patients "unmask" or experience symptoms due their body's rapid shift in response to their second or third shots or sometimes later shots. The second situation is when a very mixed diet is required to control post-shot hypersensitivity symptoms.

If your doctor suspects you are unmasking, he or she may give you a handout about Dr. McEwen's VMD which explains how it works as well as giving the formulas for the food mixtures Dr. McEwen prescribes for his unmasking patients to eat. If you do not have the handout, a little explanation here might be helpful.

The basic principle behind the VMD is that for every allergen, there is a particular dose of the allergen that causes the maximum reaction. A larger dose, especially if it is eaten at four or five day intervals in a rotation diet, will not cause symptoms. (Thus, foods that we consider our safest foods because we eat them on a rotation diet without problems are not actually foods that we are not allergic to). If one were to graph the strength of an allergic reaction versus the dose of the allergen, the graph would be a curve with a high point in the middle and low points (no symptoms) at both the high and low ends of the dosage scale. On a rotation diet, we are eating an amount of the food that is "above" the peak of the tolerance curve. As treatment progresses, the curve shifts to the right. Now the amount of food we were eating without symptoms is in the part of the curve that is the highest on the strength of the reaction. Thus, the solution is to eat on the other end of the curve – to eat foods in very small quantities. In order to get enough to eat, you will need to eat several to many foods at each meal (I was told that nine was the minimum number) in very small amounts. As the shot "ripens" or, for some patients, with subsequent shots., the reaction high point of the tolerance curve moves farther toward the high end of the dosage scale, and normal-sized servings of the food will be tolerated without causing symptoms once again.

For any allergen – inhalant, food, or chemical – LDA or EPD treatment does not eliminate your allergy to that substance. What it does is make the dosage required to provoke a reaction 10 to 1000 times higher than the dosage that caused symptoms before the patient began taking low dose immunotherapy shots.

The VMD, as it was originally developed by Dr. Len McEwen, is based on a specific set of fairly common foods. Many EPD and LDA patients I have talked to who have been put on the VMD by their doctors react to one of more of the standard VMD mixtures. The grain mixture is usually the most problematic, followed by the meat mixture. Therefore, these patients must find other "safe" foods to substitute for the foods they are reacting to in the standard mixtures, or they may need to "start from scratch" and eat many rare or exotic foods that they have not eaten much in the past in 1 teaspoon to 1 tablespoon amounts at each meal. Thus, they are following the principles of the VMD rather than the specific details of Dr. McEwen's VMD. For more about this type of VMD, see the next chapter.

Using the VMD for unmasking is a balancing act, and the balance can change from day to day as your shot ripens or wanes. However, with subsequent shots, you should reach a stable place. In the meantime, do not get discouraged. Do not be concerned if you cannot follow Dr. McEwen's VMD as written, or even the VMD that seemed to work for you a few days ago without reaction. If you can add more foods, thus eating each food in smaller quantities, that is one way to improve your tolerance for the VMD. Another variation on the VMD that may lessen your reactions is Dr. Shrader's "crazy rotation" which is described in the LDA patient instruction book. It is basically having at least three sets of at least nine foods, and eating one set of foods in VMD quantities for all meals on day one, the second set on day 2, and the third set on day 3 of your crazy rotation cycle.

For more tips on using the VMD and for improving your tolerance for it, see pages 46 and 70 to 71.

Your Personal Very Mixed Diet

This chapter contains ideas that you can use as a springboard for devising your own personalized VMD. Be sure to discuss these ideas with your doctor before implementing them.

I have used a personalized "exotic" VMD for a few weeks around my shots (not including the critical three days, during which I use a glycerin solution) for years as a way to deal with post-shot hypersensitivity. Because I may begin reacting to a formerly "safe" food after using it at shot time for several shots, and also because the foods I eat are so exotic that I can't buy more easily on the spur of the moment, I never mix the foods. Instead, I put a small (less than 1 tablespoon) amount of each separate food on a plate, cover it with paper towel, and microwave it to make my meals. By eating this way, if I seem to be reacting to my meals, I can remove foods one at a time until I find the offending food. Then all that is wasted is that one food, not everything I was planning to eat.

This is a pretty boring way to eat, I admit. I have talked to satisfied VMD users who make crock pot stew using several types of game meat and a dozen or more vegetables. They eat this every day for every meal, but find it more appealing than small bits of food arranged separately on a plate.

The bottom line advice for those of you who are working out your own VMD or other around-shot-time diet (such as eating exotic, page 38) is two-fold: (1) Eat all foods in small quantities and eat as many foods as possible to avoid reactions and sensitizing to new foods, and (2) As Dr. Shrader told me years ago, "Do whatever works." Each of us is an individual with unique allergies and reactions. You are the only one who can ferret out what foods might be causing you problems. Talk to your doctor (who might tell you "Do whatever works") and then experiment, keeping the quantity of each food small, until you find what works best for you. Keep in mind that if you are using the VMD for unmasking, you WILL get through it sooner than you might think.

The next four chapters contain information about and recipes for Dr. Len McEwen's VMD and can also contribute ideas for your own personalized VMD.

Very Mixed Non-Grain Flour Mixture

If you have difficulty tolerating the grain mixture on Dr. McEwen's VMD, this non-grain mixture might be a substitute for you. The flours from Special Foods (see "Sources," page 82) used in this mixture are not as uniform in texture as grain flours and can vary from batch to batch, so if you have a scale, it may be best to measure your flours for mixing by weight rather than by volume. If you do not have a scale, the volumes below will give you approximately equal weights of the last six flours with a double weight of arrowroot.

2 cups arrowroot
1 cup amaranth flour
1 cup cassava flour
1 cup malanga flour
⅞ cup lotus flour
¾ cup white sweet potato flour
¾ cup true yam flour

Stir each type of flour before measuring it. Measure the flours into a large bowl and stir them together thoroughly. Use in the following recipes or store any leftover flour for future use. Makes about 2⅛ pounds flour mixture.

Mixed Exotic Tortillas

2 cups non-grain flour mixture, above
¼ teaspoon salt
⅞ to 1 cup boiling water, cooled slightly

Combine the flour and salt. Add the water and stir and knead to form a dough about the consistency of Play-doh™. Divide the dough into 12 portions. Roll and cook as directed in the "Shot-Time Diet Tortillas" recipe on page 19. Makes 12 tortillas.

Mixed Exotic Muffins

2 cups non-grain flour mixture, page 47
¼ teaspoon salt
1 teaspoon baking soda
1 teaspoon cream of tartar OR 3 teaspoons rhubarb concentrate, page 36
1 cup water
2 tablespoons oil, possibly a mixture of oils that you usually tolerate

Oil and flour the cups of a muffin tin, or use paper liners. Mix the flour, salt, baking soda, and cream of tartar (if you are using it) in a large bowl. Combine the water, oil, and rhubarb concentrate (if you are using it) and stir them into the flour mixture. Put the batter in the prepared muffin tin, filling the cups about ¾ full. Bake at 350°F for 25 to 30 minutes. (They will not brown very much). Makes 10 muffins.

Mixed Exotic Pancakes

1 cup non-grain flour mixture, page 47
¼ teaspoon salt
½ teaspoon baking soda
½ teaspoon cream of tartar or 1½ teaspoons rhubarb concentrate, page 36
⅞ cup water
1 tablespoon oil

Lightly oil your pancake griddle and begin heating it over medium heat or to 350°F if you are using an electric griddle. Mix the flour, salt, baking soda, and cream of tartar (if you are using it) in a large bowl. Combine the water, oil, and rhubarb concentrate (if you are using it) and stir them into the flour mixture. Pour about ⅛ cup batter onto the griddle for each pancake and cook until it is dry on the top and brown on the bottom. Turn and cook the other side, also allowing it to brown thoroughly. (If these pancakes are not very thoroughly cooked, they tend to be gooey inside, but reheating in a toaster-oven helps this problem). If the batter thickens while you are cooking the pancakes, add 1 to 2 tablespoons more water to return it to the right consistency for pancakes. Makes about 1 dozen pancakes which freeze well.

Mixed Exotic Burger Buns

Make muffins, page 48, except bake them in an oiled and floured Texas-size muffin pan or 6 oiled and floured custard cups. When cool, slice horizontally with a serrated knife. Makes 6 buns.

Mixed Exotic Cookies

1 cup non-grain flour mixture, page 47
¼ teaspoon baking soda
¼ teaspoon cream of tartar or ¾ teaspoon rhubarb concentrate, page 36
¼ cup Fruit Sweet™ (See "Sources," page 78).
¼ cup oil, possibly a mixture of oils that you tolerate

Combine the flour, baking soda, and cream of tartar (if you are using it) in a bowl. Mix together the Fruit Sweet™, oil, and rhubarb concentrate (if you are using it) and stir them into the flour mixture. Drop by heaping teaspoons on an oiled baking sheet and flatten them with oiled fingers held together. Bake at 375°F for 8 to 10 minutes or until lightly browned. Makes about 1½ dozen cookies.

Mixed Less-Allergenic Vegetables

1 cup sliced carrots
1 cup sliced fennel or celery
1 cup water
½ teaspoon salt
1¼ cups halved and sliced summer squash, such as crookneck
1 cup peeled, seeded, and cubed winter squash, such as butternut
    (butternut gets less mushy than some of the other kinds)
1½ cups thawed frozen artichoke hearts, cut into quarters

Choose four or more of the above vegetables. Combine the carrots, celery or fennel, water, and salt in a saucepan. Bring to a boil and cook 10 minutes. Add the rest of the vegetables and cook another 5 to 10 minutes, or until very tender. Makes 6 to 8 servings.

Mixed Dried Fruit Snack

This mixture is handy to carry along when you are away from home if you tolerate it. (See the note below).

Combine ¾ cup quartered dried peach halves, 1 cup halved dried apple slices, 1 cup dried banana pieces, ½ cup raisins, and ½ cup sugar-free dried blueberries. Makes about 4 cups of fruit snack.

Note: It is not advisable to eat one VMD mixture alone. Carry along a muffin, some cold meat, etc. to have with this. Also, dried fruit (or for some patients, any fruit) may be a problem for patients with *Candida* and should be eliminated completely around shot time.

Dr. McEwen's Very Mixed Diet

Dr. Len McEwen originally wrote his VMD to help patients who were "unmasking" after their second or third shots. I heard him giving a lecture on a tape where he told a humorous anecdote about himself, as a non-cook, devising and writing his VMD while waiting in an airport! Dr. McEwen's VMD is based on a specific set of foods, some of which may be problematic for highly food-allergic low dose immunotherapy patients. If you find that the food mixtures used in the next four chapters cause symptoms, you may do better eating mixtures of other foods instead, possibly including rare foods. See the previous two chapters for more information about this and discuss developing your own VMD with your doctor.

The VMD mixture recipes in this chapter simplify the cooking process and Americanize of some of the basic mixtures contained in Dr. McEwen's very mixed diet. The mixtures below are used in the recipes found in the next three chapters.

Very Mixed Diet Flour Mixture

Dr. McEwen's VMD flour mixture specifies weights and was designed for the average English kitchen equipped with a scale. However, we Americans don't always own one. Since the weights of the various flours below are almost exactly the same (1 cup of each flour weighs within 0.1 ounce of 4.5 ounces), I find it easier to make up the VMD flour mixture using measuring cups rather than a scale.

1 cup barley flour
1 cup rye flour
1 cup rice flour
1 cup millet flour
1 cup garbanzo (chick pea) flour
2 cup buckwheat flour
2 cup sago or tapioca* flour

Stir each type of flour before measuring it. Measure the flours into a large bowl, and stir them together thoroughly. Use this flour mixture in the recipes in the next chapter or store any leftover flour for future use. Makes about 2½ pounds of flour mixture.

*NOTE: I do not know of any source for sago. However, having a sticky starch as a part of this flour mixture improves its baking properties. I asked Dr. Shrader if it would be all right to use tapioca in place of the sago because tapioca is a part of the very mixed diet in the potato mixture, and his answer was, "Yes."

Easy Baked Very Mixed Diet Grain Mixture

Dr. McEwen's VMD suggests boiling the VMD grains separately and then mixing them. Timing is not as critical when grains are cooked in the oven, and this method of preparing them makes less mess in the kitchen. Also, long, slow cooking makes the whole grains easier to digest. If you are preparing all of the VMD mixtures, bake this with the fish mixture on page 53 and potato mixture on page 54.

1½ ounces (¼ cup minus ½ tablespoon) pearled barley
1½ ounces (¼ cup) rye
5¾ to 6 cups water
1 teaspoon salt, or to taste
3 ounces (½ cup) buckwheat
1½ ounces (¼ cup) brown rice
1½ ounces (¼ cup) lentils
1½ ounces (¼ cup minus 1 teaspoon) millet

Combine the barley and rye with 5¾ cups water and the salt in a 3-quart glass casserole dish with a lid. Bake at 350°F for one hour. Stir in the buckwheat, rice, and lentils and bake for another hour. Stir in the millet and bake for an additional ½ hour, or until all of the grains are soft and the water is absorbed. Check occasionally as the end of the baking time approaches, adding more water if necessary. Makes about 5 cups cooked grains, or 8 to 12 servings.

Very Mixed Diet Fish Mixture

½ pound cod
½ pound skate (See note on skate, page 71).
½ pound salmon
Water
½ teaspoon salt, or to taste

Put the fish in a glass baking dish in a single layer and add water to a depth of ½ inch. Sprinkle with the salt. Cover the dish with its lid or foil and bake at 350°F for 20 to 25 minutes or until the fish is opaque throughout and flakes easily with a fork. (If the fish is of different thicknesses and some of it cooks more quickly, remove the ones that are done first and leave the rest in the oven to finish cooking). Cool slightly. Strain and reserve the cooking liquid. Remove the bones and skin and flake the fish. Mix together the different types of flaked fish and use in the recipes on page 63.

Very Mixed Diet Ground Meat Mixture

½ pound or 1 cup ground beef
½ pound or 1 cup ground lamb
½ pound or 1 cup ground pork
½ pound or 1 cup ground venison
½ pound or 1 cup ground chicken (about 2 thighs plus one leg or
    ¾ whole breast required)
½ pound or 1 cup ground rabbit (about 2 hind legs required)

Choose at least four of the meats above. If some of the meat you wish to use, such as chicken or rabbit, is not ground when purchased, cut it off the bone, cut it into 1 inch cubes, and freeze it overnight. (See note on boning meats, page 71). Thaw it partially and put the cubes in a food processor or blender. "Pulse" until the meat is ground. (If you do not have a processor or blender, mince finely with a knife or scissors). Combine the ground meats, using your hands to mix them thoroughly. Use in the recipes on pages 60 to 62.

Very Mixed Diet Mixed Vegetables

2 cups sliced carrots
1 cup sliced celery
1 cup cut green beans, fresh or frozen
1 cup water
½ teaspoon salt
1 cup peas, fresh or frozen

Combine the carrots, celery, beans, water, and salt in a saucepan. Bring to a boil and cook 10 minutes. Add the peas, return to a boil, and cook another 5 minutes, or until tender. Makes 6 to 8 servings.

Very Mixed Diet Potato Mixture

2 large (about 10 ounces each) white potatoes
2 large (about 10 ounces each) sweet potatoes
½ cup granulated tapioca or small pearl tapioca
2 cups water
½ teaspoon salt, or to taste

Bake the white and sweet potatoes at 400°F for 1 hour or at 350°F for 1½ hours or until they feel soft when squeezed. Combine the water and tapioca in a saucepan. (This produces approximately "equal" portions of white potatoes, sweet potatoes, and fresh tapioca). Let the pearl tapioca stand overnight or the granulated tapioca stand for at least 5 minutes. Bring the mixture to a boil. Boil the granulated tapioca one minute, remove it from the heat, and allow it to stand for at least 20 minutes. Boil the pearl tapioca for 5 to 10 minutes, or until most of the pearls of tapioca are clear. Peel the potatoes. Add them and the salt to the tapioca mixture and mash. Makes 6 to 8 servings.

Very Mixed Diet Fruit Mixture

1 cup peeled, chopped apple (about 1 large or 1½ small)

1 cup dried banana pieces

1 cup blackberries, fresh or frozen

½ cup raisins

3 cups rhubarb slices

1 cup peeled, chopped peaches (about 1 large or 1½ small fresh peaches, or use frozen peaches)

1 cup water

2 to 4 tablespoons fructose* (optional – omit this if you are allergic to corn)

⅛ teaspoon cinnamon (optional)

Mix together the water, raisins, and banana pieces in a saucepan and begin cooking them over medium heat while you peel and chop the apples, peaches, and rhubarb. Add the rest of the fruit and cook until it is tender, about 25-30 minutes total cooking time. Add cinnamon and fructose to taste. (*Fructose is usually made from corn. If you are corn sensitive, omit the fructose). Makes about 5½ to 6 cups of fruit mixture.

Very Mixed Diet Baked Goods

VMD Crackers

3 cups VMD flour mixture, page 51

1 teaspoon baking soda

1 teaspoon salt (optional)

1 teaspoon cream of tartar OR 1 tablespoon rhubarb concentrate, page 36

1 cup water

¼ cup oil, possibly a mixture of oils you tolerate

Combine the flour, baking soda, salt, and cream of tartar (if you are using it) in a large bowl. Mix together the water, oil, and rhubarb concentrate (if you are using it) and pour them into the flour mixture. Stir until the dough sticks together, adding another tablespoon or two of water if needed to form a stiff but not crumbly dough. Divide the dough in half. Roll each half to about ⅛ inch thickness on a lightly oiled cookie sheet using a lightly oiled rolling pin. Cut into 2 inch squares. Sprinkle the tops of the crackers lightly with additional salt if desired. Bake at 375°F for 15 to 20 minutes, or until the crackers are crisp and lightly browned. Makes 6 to 7 dozen crackers.

VMD Pancakes

2 cups VMD flour mixture, page 51

½ teaspoon salt

1 teaspoon baking soda

1 teaspoon cream of tartar OR 3 teaspoons rhubarb concentrate, page 36

1¾ cups water

2 tablespoons oil, possibly a mixture of oils you tolerate

Lightly oil your pancake griddle and begin heating it over medium heat or to 350°F if you are using an electric griddle. Mix the flour, salt, baking soda, and cream of tartar (if you are using it) in a large bowl. Combine the water, oil, and rhubarb concentrate (if you are using it) and stir them into the flour mixture. Pour about ⅛ cup batter onto the griddle for each pancake and cook until dry on the top. Turn and cook the other side. (These pancakes do not brown much). If the batter thickens while you are cooking the pancakes, add more water to return it to the right consistency for pancakes. Makes about 1½ to 2 dozen pancakes which freeze well.

VMD Muffins

2 cups VMD flour mixture, page 51
¼ teaspoon salt (optional)
1 teaspoon baking soda
1 teaspoon cream of tartar OR 3 teaspoons rhubarb concentrate, page 36
1 cup water
2 tablespoons oil, possibly a mixture of oils you tolerate

Oil and flour the cups of a muffin tin or use paper liners. Mix the flour, salt, baking soda, and cream of tartar (if you are using it) in a large bowl. Combine the water, oil, and rhubarb concentrate (if you are using it) and stir them into the flour mixture. Put the batter in the prepared muffin tin, filling the cups about ¾ full. Bake at 350°F for 20 to 25 minutes. (The muffins will not brown very much). Makes 11 to 12 muffins.

VMD Tortillas

2 cups VMD flour mixture, page 51
½ teaspoon salt
¾ cup water

Stir together the flour and salt. Add the water and stir and knead to form a dough about the consistency of Play-doh™. Divide the dough into 6 to 8 portions. Flour each portion well and roll it out to about ⅛ inch thickness on a well floured board, turning the dough over and flouring it on both sides while rolling it. Heat a heavy frying pan over medium heat. (Add no oil). One at a time, put each tortilla into the pan and cook it for 2 to 3 minutes on the first side, or until it begins to brown in spots on the underside. Turn it with a spatula and cook it for 2 to 3 minutes on the second side also. (If you are not sensitive to coatings such as teflon, an electric tortilla maker is an easy and quick way to make these tortillas. See "Sources," page 82). Cool the tortillas on a dishtowel or a wire rack. Makes 6 to 8 tortillas.

VMD No-Yeast Bread

4 cups VMD flour mixture, page 51
¾ teaspoon salt
2 teaspoons baking soda
2 teaspoons cream of tartar OR 2 tablespoons rhubarb
    concentrate, page 36
2 cups water
¼ cup oil, possibly a mixture of oils you tolerate

Oil and flour a 9 by 5 inch loaf pan. Mix the flour, salt, baking soda, and cream of tartar (if you are using it) in a large bowl. Combine the water, oil, and rhubarb concentrate (if you are using it) and stir them into the flour mixture. Put the batter in the prepared pan. Bake at 350°F for 40 to 50 minutes. (The bread will not brown very much). Place the loaf on a rack and cool it completely before slicing. Makes 1 loaf.

VMD Yeast Bread

1¾ cups warm (105-115°F) water
4 tablespoons apple juice concentrate, thawed
1½ packages (3¾ teaspoons) active dry yeast
3 tablespoons oil, possibly a mixture of oils you tolerate
1 teaspoon salt
4 teaspoons guar gum
6 to 6½ cups VMD flour mixture, page 51

Mix the water with the juice in a large electric mixer bowl. Stir in the yeast and allow the mixture to stand for about 10 minutes or until it is foamy. Add the oil and salt to the yeast mixture. Stir the guar gum into half of the flour and add this mixture to the liquid ingredients in the mixer bowl. Beat at medium speed for three minutes. Mix in the rest of the flour with the mixer and your hands and knead the dough on a floured board for 5 to 10 minutes. Shape the dough into a loaf and put it in an oiled 8 by 4 inch or 9 by 5 inch loaf pan. Place the loaf in a warm (85°F to 90°F) place and allow it to rise for 40 to 50 minutes, or until the dough is to the top of the pan. Bake at 375°F for 50 to 60 minutes, or until it is light brown. Place the loaf on a rack and cool it completely before slicing. Makes one loaf.

VMD Sandwich Buns

For no-yeast buns, make VMD muffins, page 57, except bake them in 6 large glass custard cups instead of a muffin tin. If you allow them to brown well on the bottom, they will be less likely to fall apart when you slice them and use them for a sandwich.

For yeast buns, make VMD yeast bread dough, above. Shape the dough into 10 to 12 balls and place them on a lightly oiled baking sheet. Let rise again in a warm place until double, about 30 minutes. Bake at 375°F for 25 to 30 minutes. (These buns will not brown very much). Makes 10 to 12 sandwich buns.

Very Mixed Diet Main and Side Dishes

VMD Stroganoff

¾ pound VMD meat mixture, page 53
1 cup water
2 tablespoons VMD flour mixture, page 51
½ to 1 teaspoon salt, or to taste
Cooked VMD noodles, below, or VMD grain mixture, page 52

Brown the meat in a skillet. Shake together the water and flour in a glass jar and add them to the meat. Cook, stirring, until the mixture thickens and boils. Boil at least one minute. Season with salt to taste and serve over noodles or grains. Makes 3 to 4 servings.

VMD Noodles

½ cup water
1 tablespoon oil, possibly a mixture of oils you tolerate
1¼ to 1½ cups VMD flour mixture, page 51, divided
Water
Salt

Mix ½ cup water and the oil in a bowl. Add 1 cup of the flour and beat it with a fork for 1 to 2 minutes. Knead in enough of the remaining flour to make a soft but not sticky dough. Roll it on a well floured board to between $\frac{1}{16}$ and $\frac{1}{8}$ inch in thickness. Leaving the dough flat (do not roll it up, or it will break), cut the dough into noodles with a long knife. Bring about 3 quarts of salted water to a boil. Add the noodles and cook until *al dente*, about 2 to 4 minutes.

If you make these often, you may wish to purchase a spaetlze press. After making and kneading the dough, above, rinse the press with cold water. Bring about 3 quarts of salted water to a boil. Put the dough in the press, hold it a few inches above the boiling water, and press out the noodles. After the noodles rise to the surface, boil them an additional ½ to 1 minute. Taste them to see if they are done; do not overcook.

When the noodles are cooked, drain them immediately in a colander and serve them with a little oil and salt, with stroganoff, page 60, or in soup, below. Makes 2 to 4 servings.

VMD Meatballs or Burgers

1 pound (2 cups) VMD meat mixture, page 53
¾ teaspoon salt, or to taste

Mix the meat with the salt and form it into meatballs or four burgers. To cook meatballs, rub a skillet with a little fat from one of the meats you are using, if available. Cook the meatballs until brown on all sides in the skillet. For burgers, broil for 10 minutes on each side and serve on buns, page 59. Makes 4 servings.

VMD Soup

1 pound (2 cups) VMD meat mixture, page 53
1½ teaspoons salt, divided
⅔ cup sliced carrots
⅓ cup peas, fresh or frozen
⅓ cup cut green beans, fresh or frozen
⅓ cup sliced celery
8 cups (2 quarts) water
Cooked VMD noodles, page 60 or VMD grain mixture, page 52
    (optional)

Prepare small meatballs as in the recipe above using the meat and ½ teaspoon salt. Brown them in a stockpot. Pour off the fat and add the remaining ingredients except the noodles. Simmer for 1 to 1½ hours, adding the noodles the last few minutes. Makes 6 servings.

VMD Meatloaf or Burgers

1 pound (2 cups) VMD meat mixture, page 53
¾ cup VMD mixed vegetables, page 54, drained
½ cup VMD grain mixture, page 52
¾ teaspoon salt, or to taste
¼ cup water (for meatloaf only)

Put the vegetables, grains, and salt in a food processor or blender and puree briefly. (It is all right if some chunks remain). Remove the vegetable mixture from the processor or blender, combine it with the meat with your hands, and form into a loaf. Place it in a 2- to 3-quart casserole dish with the water. Cover the dish with its lid and bake at 350°F for 45 minutes. Uncover and bake for another 20 minutes, or until the meatloaf is brown. To make burgers, form the meat-vegetable mixture into 6 patties and broil for 10 minutes on each side. Serve with buns, page 59. Makes 4 to 6 servings.

VMD Swiss Steak

1 pound (2 cups) VMD meat mixture, page 53
1 teaspoon salt, divided, or to taste
1 cup water
½ tablespoon VMD flour mixture, page 51

Mix the meat with ½ teaspoon salt and form four patties. Pan fry until brown on both sides, remove from the pan, and pour off any fat. Shake the water, flour, and remaining salt together in a jar and add to the pan. Cook, stirring, until the gravy thickens and boils. Boil for 1 minute; then return the meat to the pan and heat through. Makes 4 servings.

Kedgeree

2 cups VMD grain mixture, page 52
2 cups VMD fish mixture, page 53
1 cup water or fish cooking liquid, page 53
2 tablespoons VMD flour mixture, page 51
½ teaspoon salt, or to taste
1 hard boiled egg*, chopped, if tolerated

Shake the water or fish liquid, flour, and salt together in a jar. Transfer to a saucepan and cook over medium heat until it thickens and boils. Boil one minute. Stir in the grains and fish and heat, stirring often, until just heated through. Serve garnished with the chopped egg, if desired. Makes 4 to 6 servings.

*Although hard for Americans to believe, the British dish kedgeree, made with egg, is so favored by the British that it is a part of Dr. McEwen's VMD! If you are allergic to eggs (one of the most "potent" food allergens), omit the egg garnish.

"Creamed" Fish

2 cups water or fish cooking liquid, page 53
5 tablespoons VMD flour mixture, page 51
1 teaspoon salt, or to taste
1 to 1½ cups VMD fish mixture, page 53
VMD bread, muffins, pancakes, or tortillas pages 56 to 59,
    VMD grain mixture, page 52, or VMD noodles, page 60

Shake the water or fish liquid, flour, and salt together in a jar. Transfer to a saucepan and cook over medium heat until it thickens and boils. Boil one minute. Stir in the fish and heat, stirring often, until the fish is heated through. Serve over bread, muffins, pancakes, tortillas, or warm grain mixture or noodles. Makes 4 servings.

Very Mixed Diet Desserts and Snacks

VMD Cobbler

¼ cup water

2 tablespoons tapioca

3 cups (about ½ batch) VMD fruit mixture, page 55

¾ cup VMD flour mixture, page 51

¾ teaspoon baking soda

¾ teaspoon cream of tartar OR 2 ¼ teaspoons rhubarb
    concentrate, page 36

¼ cup water

1 tablespoon oil, possibly a mixture of oils you tolerate

Combine ¼ cup water and the tapioca in a saucepan and let stand for 5 minutes. Add the fruit mixture and bring to a boil. Put the fruit into a 2 to 3-quart casserole dish. In a bowl, stir together the flour, baking soda, and cream of tartar, if you are using it. Combine ¼ cup water, the oil, and the rhubarb concentrate (if you are using it) and stir them into the flour mixture until just mixed. Put on top of the fruit and bake at 350°F 25 to 30 minutes or until brown. Makes 6 servings.

VMD Sorbet

Freeze very mixed diet fruit mixture, page 55, in ice cube trays overnight. Remove from the freezer and allow them to soften at room temperature for 20 to 30 minutes. Put 2 cubes in a blender or food processor and process until smooth. Add cubes one at a time, processing after each addition, until all the cubes have been added. One batch of very mixed diet fruit mixture makes about 6 cups of sorbet.

VMD Cookies

2¼ cups VMD flour mixture, page 51
1 teaspoon baking soda
1½ cups VMD fruit mixture, page 55
¼ cup oil, possibly a mixture of oils you tolerate

Mix flour and baking soda. Puree the fruit mixture in a food processor or blender; add the oil and process a few more seconds. Stir the fruit and oil into the flour and soda until just mixed. Drop by heaping teaspoons on an oiled baking sheet and flatten them with your oiled fingers held together. Bake at 350°F for 15 to 20 minutes, or until lightly browned. Makes about 3 dozen cookies.

Purple Cupcakes

2 cups VMD flour mixture, page 51
1 teaspoon baking soda
2 cups VMD fruit mixture, page 55
¼ cup oil, possibly a mixture of oils you tolerate

Mix flour and baking soda. Puree the fruit mixture in a food processor or blender; add the oil and process a few more seconds. Stir the fruit and oil into the flour and soda until just mixed. Fill oiled and floured or paper-lined muffin cups ¾ full with the batter and bake at 350°F for 30 to 35 minutes, or until a toothpick inserted in the center comes out clean. Makes about 12 cupcakes.

VMD Jam or Purple Frosting

1 tablespoon water
1 tablespoon tapioca flour
1 cup VMD fruit mixture, page 55

Combine the water and tapioca flour in a saucepan. Puree the fruit mixture with a blender or food processor. Stir it into the tapioca mixture thoroughly. Cook over medium heat until it thickens and boils, stirring often. Use to frost "Purple Cupcakes," above, or as jam on bread, muffins, or crackers, pages 56 to 59.

VMD Pretzels

½ batch "VMD Yeast Bread" dough, page 59
Salt, coarse if available without additives

Make dough for "VMD Yeast Bread" as directed in the recipe. Divide it into 16 pieces and roll each piece into a 12 to 15 inch long rope. Place the ropes on lightly oiled baking sheets and shape them into pretzel (open knot) shapes. Brush them lightly with cold water and sprinkle them with coarse salt. Allow them to rise in a warm place for about 30 minutes. Bake at 350°F for 20 to 25 minutes, or until they are set and lightly browned on the bottom. Remove them from the baking sheet immediately with a metal spatula and cool them on a wire rack. Makes 16 3 to 4-inch pretzels.

Notes and Tips

On leavening: Non-yeast baked goods are leavened by mixing an acid component, such as vitamin C crystals, with a basic component, such as baking soda. For three weeks after an injection, low dose immunotherapy patients must restrict their intake of vitamin C to 500 mg per day. Therefore, they must either keep track of how much vitamin C they are consuming in baked goods and stop eating them when they reach their vitamin C limit, or they should use a substitute acid component for leavening, such as cream of tartar, rhubarb concentrate, lemon juice, or lime juice (if tolerated).

To substitute cream of tartar for vitamin C powder or crystals, an approximate rule of thumb is to use 1 to 1½ times the amount of baking soda called for in the recipe. For example, if your recipe calls for 1 teaspoon baking soda and ¼ teaspoon vitamin C, use 1 teaspoon baking soda and 1 to 1½ teaspoons cream of tartar. Mix the cream of tartar with the dry ingredients. If the recipe contains fruit, slightly less cream of tartar may be required. Cream of tartar is highly purified potassium bitartrate crystals. Its manufacture begins with a byproduct from wine-making. Because of its purity, it usually does not cause problems, but patients who are highly sensitive to grapes or brewer's yeast may want to keep its original source in mind and use rhubarb concentrate for the acid component of the leavening process instead.

To substitute rhubarb concentrate (recipe on page 36) or, if you are not allergic to citrus fruits, lemon juice or lime juice for vitamin C crystals, a rule of thumb is to use three times the amount of baking soda called for in the recipe. For example, if your recipe calls for 1 teaspoon baking soda and ¼ teaspoon vitamin C, use 1 teaspoon baking soda and 3 teaspoons rhubarb concentrate, lemon juice, or lime juice. Mix the rhubarb concentrate or lemon or lime juice with the liquid ingredients. The amount of other liquids may need to be decreased in the same amount as the liquid leavening that you add. If the recipe contains fruit, slightly less rhubarb concentrate, lemon juice, or lime juice may be required.

On using fructose or glycerin rather than the shot-time diet: Patients who are sensitive to all or almost all of the foods on the shot-time diet may be advised by their doctors to use a fructose or glycerin solution rather than the shot-time diet around the time of their shot. Glycerin is metabolized like a fat and fructose is metabolized more slowly than other types of sugars, so they should not cause major swings in blood sugar levels like sugar can. My personal experience with using the fructose and glycerin solutions was that it is not as difficult as I had expected it to be. Mixing the fructose or glycerin with hot water may be more satisfying than drinking the solution cold. Or you can make "slush" by mixing ¼ cup of bottled water with 4 teaspoons fructose or glycerin in a food processor and adding a tray of bottled water ice cubes one at a time until all are finely blended. It is advisable to eat lightly when you return to eating after being on the fructose or glycerin.

On margarines that were used on the EPD diet: Two types of margarine, Granose™ and Tomor™, are allowed on the EPD diet. In the 1990s, Klaire Labs, the makers of Vital Life™ vitamins, imported Granose™ margarine from England for use by American EPD patients. After the FDA shut down EPD in 2001, Klaire Labs stopped importing it. When LDA became available, several small American companies looked into the possibility of importing Granose™ margarine again but found that they would have to import so much that they did not have the facilities to store it frozen until it was sold. However, there are distributors who will sell Tomor™ margarine in smaller quantities and it is possible that it could be imported by a small company in the future. Therefore, the recipes developed in the early 1990s which included the margarines which are acceptable on the EPD diet have been left in this book with options added for making the recipe without the margarine.

On keeping yourself from using lotions, cosmetics, etc. without thinking around the time of your shot: Keep a small brown bag in the cabinet under your kitchen and bathroom sinks. Before your shot, remove hand lotion, soaps, makeup, toothpaste, etc.

from their usual storage places and place them in the bag. After your shot, store your Magick Botanicals™ or Simple™ soap and shampoo, baking soda for brushing your teeth, etc. in the bag, where they will be all ready to go for your next shot.

On newspapers and glossy magazines: The evening of two days before our shot, we remove all newspapers and most magazines from our house. We put the TV schedule and any magazines that we do not want to throw away in well-sealed plastic bags.

On cleaning products: It is important to use the proper cleaning products and equipment when you clean before your shot. You are not helping yourself if you remove the dust and mold from your environment but leave toxic chemical residues in their place! Always use unscented products such as Bon Ami™ and SuperClean™ (see "Sources," page 80) for general cleaning. To eliminate mold, use a citrus extract product such as NutriBiotic™ ("Sources," page 80). You can dilute it 30-60 drops to 32 ounces water (or ¼ to ½ teaspoon NutriBiotic™ to 32 ounces water, rinsing the spoon into the water) in a spray bottle and use it to spray down showers, etc. To leave a stronger anti-fungal residue on the inside of your refrigerator, put several drops on a barely damp cloth and use that side of the cloth to wipe down the refrigerator walls. If you are allergic to dust, you may want to consider getting a vacuum cleaner which filters the air before returning it to your environment.

On garbage disposals: Garbage disposals are never completely free of bits of the food that has been ground in them. Bacteria and mold can easily use this food to support their growth, especially in warm climates or at a warm time of the year. Before your shot, see if there is a moldy smell after pouring boiling water in the disposal side of your sink. If you do detect this smell, or if your house is warm, clean your garbage disposal with natural cleaners in this way: First, mix some dish soap and warm water. Dip an old toothbrush in it and brush the back side of the rubber splash guard at the top of your garbage disposal. You may notice black "crud" on the toothbrush. If so, rinse the toothbrush, dip it in the soap solution, and scrub the splash guard again, repeating until the toothbrush is clean after scrubbing. Cut a lemon in half. Throw a handful of baking soda and the cut lemon in the garbage disposal and grind them down.

On polishing furniture: I prefer to polish furniture with lemon oil during non-shot months, but if you feel you must use something on your furniture close to the time of your shot and your doctor allows you to, use an all-natural, non-petrochemical product like pure lemon oil. (See "Sources," page 81).

Tips for improving your tolerance of the very mixed diet: When the very mixed diet is used to deal with "unmasking," the amount of each food in the mixtures eaten is important. You may find that you react less if you eat several mini-meals of the very mixed diet per day rather than eating three more normal-sized meals. If you use a small dish for your mini-meals and it is fairly full, you won't get the feeling of being deprived that you may get from seeing very small amounts of several mixtures on a regular-sized dish. Also, the greater number of foods or VMD mixtures you eat per meal, the better you may feel.

If you find that you do not tolerate one of the mixtures, even in very small (1 teaspoon to 1 tablespoon) amounts, you may wish to experiment with the component ingredients. With your doctor's approval, try substituting another ingredient for the one(s) you suspect may be the greatest problem for you. (However, keep in mind that Dr. Shrader says that sometimes you may need to eat small amounts of your most problematic foods to feel better). For instance, although I was allergic to all of the meats in the VMD meat mixture, beef, chicken, and venison had been more major problems for me than rabbit, pork, and lamb. When I had trouble tolerating the meat mixture, in order to have at least four meats as the diet specifies, I used pork, lamb, rabbit, and turkey, and found that I could tolerate the mixture in small amounts. Another option for a meat mixture is to substitute four ground game meats, such as kangaroo, venison, antelope, and buffalo. Another "exotic" meat mixture I have used after shots consists of a mixture of small pieces of cooked rattlesnake, alligator, and frog, which are good rolled in a mixed exotic tortilla. (See the tortilla recipe on page 47). For recipes for cooking snake, alligator, and frog, see *The Ultimate Food Allergy Cookbook and Survival Guide.* (For more information about this book, turn to the last few pages of this book). If the VMD grain mixture (page 52) or VMD flour mixture (page 51) is a problem for you, consider using the non-grain flour mixture on page 47.

Some patients make a crock pot stew of 20 to 30 of their safest vegetables and meats to eat for all of their meals after their shots. Another variation on the principles of the VMD is Dr. Shrader's "crazy rotation" which is described in the LDA patient instruction book and on page 45 of this book.

On skate and the VMD fish mixture: Although Dr. McEwen's VMD calls for skate in the fish mixture, it may be difficult or impossible for Americans to obtain skate for the VMD. In that case, with your doctor's approval, substitute a kind of fish that you do not suspect to be a major problem for you and/or that you have rarely eaten for the skate in the fish mixture.

On boning meats for the VMD: If you are using chicken or rabbit as part of your VMD meat mixture (page 53), you may be spending a lot of time boning meat. To simplify your work with chicken, call around to stores in your area; you might be able to find frozen ground chicken. If you are using rabbit, you may wish to just remove about 80% of the meat from the bones, and then bake the bones with a little water in a covered dish at 350°F for 1 to 1½ hours. Remove the rest of the meat from the bones after cooking and grind it in a food processor. Combine each 5 ounces of cooked ground rabbit with 8 ounces of each of the other meat you are using. Proceed with your recipes as if all of the meats were raw. If you are really pressed for time, you can cook the whole rabbit, remove all of the meat after cooking, grind it, and mix it with the other meats in 5 ounces cooked to 8 ounces raw proportion.

Baking Without Special Foods™

This stop-gap revision of *The Low Dose Immunotherapy Handbook* has been necessitated by the possible demise of Special Foods™, the only source for many of the flours used in the baking recipes in this book. In 2012, the Special Foods™ website disappeared and they didn't answer their phone for about six months. They began accepting orders after that hiatus but in 2014, they again stopped answering their phone.

Ideally, I should re-do all the baking recipes now, but there is still a possibility that Special Foods™ might again reappear as it did a few years ago. My second reason for delaying a major revision of this book is that in 2014 I had viral pneumonia that went into uncontrolled asthma. One LDA shot helped some, and I'm hoping the second will bring me back to near-normal, but I'm still not physically able to do all the baking required for a major revision at this time. Therefore, I'm depending on the most amazingly resourceful allergy cook and LDA patient I've ever met, Dr. Ruth Gornet-Irwin, PhD, math professor and mother of two elementary school-age boys who take LDA. Due to the high price of Special Foods™ flours, she ground Sundial™ cassava meal with a Kitchenaid™ coffee grinder (which had never been used for coffee) and successfully used this flour in place of Special Foods™ cassava flour for the recipes in this book. Next, she found a source of commercialy ground cassava flour which is processed quickly in a way to avoid yeast growth and which works in place of Special Foods™ cassava flour in the recipes in this book. It is Otto's Naturals™ cassava flour. (See http://www.ottos naturals.com).

Ruth also has explored the problem of leavening baked goods made with Special Foods™ flours. Baking powder from Special Foods™ contained one of their flours (to match the flour you were baking with), baking soda, and calcium phosphate. Ruth has substituted baking soda plus starch-free Bakewell Cream.™ (www.new englandcupboard.com/bakewell-cream.php). The Bakewell Cream™ serves as the acid component of the leavening process and contains only acid sodium pyrophosphate. She and her sons have eaten baked goods made with starch-free Bakewell Cream™ during the week before and three weeks after their LDA shots. When asked if it was safe during the critical three days, Dr. W. A. Shrader emailed, "I can think of no reason it wouldn't be, but it hasn't been proven as I know yet." He said something very similar to me when I asked him about the Special Foods™ baking powder 23 years ago, and now that EPD and LDA patients have used them for many years without problems, they're "proven." If you try using starch-free Bakewell Cream during the critical three days, please contact me using the contact form on food-allergy.org so we can build up a body of proof for the use of starch-free Bakewell Cream™ during the critical three days.

I eventually hope to determine definite amounts of baking soda plus starch-free Bakewell Cream™ to substitute for Special Foods™ baking powders in each recipe in this book, but this will take quite a bit of baking. Until then, use the amounts Ruth has used as a starting point. They are ½ teaspoon of baking soda plus ⅓ to ½ teaspoon of starch-free Bakewell Cream™ to replace 1 teaspoon of Special Foods™ baking powder. If you notice a slight aftertaste, try decreasing the amounts. If the recipe doesn't rise, be sure you are not of overmixing; if that doesn't work, try increasing the leavening ingredients slightly. Be careful to purchase starch-free Bakewell Cream™ and not one of their products that contains corn starch.

Rhubarb concentrate is also a substitute for the acid component of baking powder and is permitted on the critical three days. Again, I cannot give absolute advice about the amounts to substitute for baking powder until I am able to do more baking. The starting point I would suggest is to use ½ teaspoon of baking soda plus 1½ teaspoons of rhubarb concentrate for 1 teaspoon of Special Foods™ baking powder. See page 67 for how to substitute rhubarb concentrate for vitamin C in leavening.

I am planning a book with all new subject matter as soon as I am able to do the cooking for it. A small taste of some of the subject matter for this book is on the next two pages. I plan to do LDA baking after that is finished and will determine definite amounts of leavening ingredients to use in the recipes in this book then if Special Foods™ is still not taking orders at that time.

Caveats for Asthma Patients

A question I am often asked by prospective low dose immuno-therapy patients is, "If these shots are so good, why hasn't my doctor heard of them?" It is because the pharmaceutical industry uses its vast financial assets and power to suppress and discredit treatments that might affect drug sales and profits, often to the detriment of the health of the American people. This is also the reason behind two very well-kept secrets about the treatment of asthma.

The first secret is that in January, 2009, the FDA banned the propellant which had been used in asthma inhalers for years ostensi-bly because it might affect the ozone layer adversely. It was replaced with hydrofluroalkane (HFA) in all propellant activated asthma inhalers and nose sprays. My local pre-EPD allergy doctor told me that when he tried to get information about what went into making HFA from the drug representatives, they didn't know anything and could give him no information. I found out why the hard way.

I had asthma when I was young but "outgrew" it and had no trouble with it until viral pneumonia brought it back last year. I was treated with inhalers which helped for a few days and then became ineffective. Then I was put on a series of more and more potent inhalers, none of which really worked. When I took an LDA shot, I had to avoid inhalers as part of the protocol. The evening of my first day without them, I felt as if a tremendous allergy burden had been lifted. The only change I had made, and had not made with previous shots, was eliminating the inhalers. I Googled "allergy to asthma inhalers" and read the experiences of bloggers who had problems with inhalers. One mother wrote about her daughter being helped by Albuterol™ administered by a nebulizer at home, but whenever she used an Albuterol™ inhaler when they were out, she got much worse. They had to rush home to stop her reaction by using the same drug with a nebulizer. Another blog told of a man whose asthma had been getting worse and his inhalers were ineffective. Then he used an old pre-propellant-change inhaler that had been stored in his hot car in an exercise bag, and it worked like magic. See page 79 for where to read these and other stories of life-threatening reactions to HFA.

The well-kept secret of asthma inhalers is that HFA is made with corn-derived ethanol. The official position is that there is not enough corn or yeast residue in HFA to cause problems. This may be true for most people, but some corn and/or yeast sensitive patients do react to the propellant. Dry powder inhalers contain lactose and traces of milk protein, so milk-allergic patients cannot use them. The only safe way to administer inhaled medications to some asthma patients is with a nebulizer. A "side effect" of the FDA mandated change in propellants is that there will be no generic inhalers for twelve to fifteen years. An online *Consumer Reports* article found that the price of non-generic inhalers nearly doubled in the first three years after the propellant change. [1]

The second well-kept secret is that there are effective natural bronchodilators that are free. One is nitrous oxide, which is in every breath taken through your nose. A second and more important natural bronchodilator is carbon dioxide (CO_2). Asthmatics lack these for two reasons: (1) many breathe mostly through their mouths, and (2) asthmatics breathe a much higher volume of air per minute, up to five or six times as much as normal people. This lowers the CO_2 level in their blood and the alveoli of their lungs which reduces the ability of hemoglobin to release oxygen into the tissues where it is needed. Over-breathing resets the CO_2 trigger that tells us when to breathe to a lower level, which perpetuates the vicious cycle of over-breathing, bronchoconstriction and asthma. The cycle can be broken by practicing the Buteyko breathing method. It is not a quick fix and requires work, discipline, and commitment, but is well worth the effort to avoid the unpleasant side effects of bronchodilator drugs. When the set-point of the trigger reaches a high enough level, under a doctor's supervision, the amount of inhaled steroids can slowly and gradually be reduced, eliminating the need for all inhalers. A full discussion of the method is beyond the scope of this book. See page 79 for sources of more information and help with the Buteyko breathing method.

[1] https://www.consumerreports.org/health/resources/pdf/best-buy-drugs/Inhaled SteroidsFINAL.pdf, page 6.

A Final Word

When I was a child, I often heard my parents quote my grand-mother, who died of cancer when I was an infant, as having often said, "When you have your health, you have everything." When you have regained your health through low dose immunotherapy, it will not have been recovered quickly or easily so don't take it for granted. Enjoy life and enjoy eating things you previously could not eat but don't become a junk food junkie and put yourself at risk for other problems. Also, use some of your newly regained energy to encourage someone who is a few shots behind you in the low dose immunother-apy process.

Sources of Special Foods and Products

Bakewell Cream™ starch-free (leavening)

New England Cupboard
PO Box 8
Hampden, ME 04444
(207) 848-4900
http://www.newenglandcupboard.com/bakewell-cream.php

Cassava, fresh (also called yucca)

Fresh cassava roots can be purchased at Safeway grocery stores and international markets. Here is the company that supplies Safeway stores, and may be able to give you information about where to get their products locally:

Sol Pacifica Products™
Progressive Produce
5790 Peachtree Street
Los Angeles, CA 90040
(800) 900-0757 or (323) 890-8100
www.progressiveproduce.com/Contact_Us.html

Cassava flour

Otto's Naturals
(732) 654-OTTO (6886) or info@ottosnaturals.com
http://www.ottosnaturals.com

Cassava meal (also called manioc flour)

Sundial Herbs
3609 Boston Road
Bronx, NY 10466
(718) 798-3962
www.sundialherbs.com

Fruit Sweet™

Wax Orchards, Inc.
P.O. Box 25448
Seattle, WA 98165
(800) 634-6132
www.waxorchards.com

Game and exotic meats

Rabbit for the 3-day diet (delicious, recently grown and
   reasonably priced)
Spring Tree Farm Rabbitry
7597 N. 67th Street
Longmont CO 80503
(720) 273-4053
http://springtreefarmsrabbitry.com/

Exotic Meats USA
1330 Capital Boulevard
Reno, Nevada, 89502
sales@exoticmeats.com
(800) 444-5687 (Russ McCurdy) or (210) 488-3729
http://www.exoticmeatsandmore.com/

Specialty Meats and Gourmet
1810 Webster Street
Hudson, Wisconsin 54016
(800) 310-2360 or (715)-386-6613
http://www.smgfoods.com/

Game Sales International, Inc.
P.O. Box 5314
Loveland, Colorado 80537
(800) 729-2090 or (303) 667-4090

Information about asthma inhalers and potentially life-threatening problems with HFA propellant

http://www.consumeraffairs.com/health/hfa_inhalers.html?page=11

http://memec08.blogspot.com/2009/07/inhaler-propellant-and-corn-allergies.html

http://cornallergygirl.com/2013/10/16/corn-free-asthma-treatment/

https://www.consumerreports.org/health/resources/pdf/best-buy-drugs/InhaledSteroidsFINAL.pdf, page 6

Information about the Buteyko Breathing Method

http://www.buteykoclinic.us/buteykoeducation.html. This page tells the history of and principles behind the Buteyko breathing method.

http://articles.mercola.com/sites/articles/archive/2013/11/24/buteyko-breathing-method.aspx. An introduction to the Buteyko breathing method with videos. Also tells how it can help with exercise and athletic pursuits.

McKeown, Patrick. *Close Your Mouth: Buteyko Clinic Handbook for Perfect Health*. Galway: Buteyko Books, 2004. This book contains all of the exercise and specifies physical conditions that make each exercise appropriate or not for you.

McKeown, Patrick. *Asthma-Free Naturally*. San Francisco: Conari Press, 2008. This book is often found in libraries but should not be used alone for self-instruction without *Close Your Mouth* or the set below because it does not contain all the exercises and precautions.

Buteyko Clinic Breathing Method 2 hour DVD, CD and Manual (*Close your Mouth*), $24.95 from Amazon. This is the best way to learn if you do not live near or cannot visit a practitioner.

http://www.buteykoclinic.us/ This website also sells the set above for a higher price, which may be worth it because the set comes with downloads and access to advice.

http://www.buteykoeducators.org/find-an-educator.html.

http://www.ncbi.nlm.nih.gov/pubmed/18951492 Medical journal article about nitric oxide production in the sinuses, which is why breathing through the nose is beneficial. In addition to the benefits mention in this abstract, nasally breathed air puts nitric oxide into the lungs where it causes bronchodilation.

http://healingnaturallybybee.com/breathing-through-your-nose-is-essential/#a5 Easy read article about benefits of nasal breathing, but do not take the large breaths it promotes if asthamtic.

Information about LDA and EPD, doctors list

www.drshrader.com

AAEM recordings of lectures about EPD and LDA

American Academy of Environmental Medicine
www.aaemonline.com
Order recordings from **lnsta-Tapes Digital Media**
(800) 669-8273
http://www.instatapes.com/online/index.htm

LDA and EPD supplies including supplements, Magick Botanicals ™ body wash and shampoo, unscented products for cleaning, dishwashing and laundry (Super-Clean™, etc.), NutriBiotic ™ anti-fungal agent, etc.

N.E.E.D.S
6666 Manlius Center Road
East Syracuse, NY 13057
1-800-634-1380
www.needs.com

Lemon oil for polishing furniture

NOW Natural Foods *(get from your health food store)*
395 S. Glen Ellyn Road
Bloomingdale, IL 60108
(800) 283-3500
www.nowfoods.com

Plastic gloves

Walter Drake, Inc.
4630 Forge Road, Suite A
Colorado Springs, CO 80907
800-525-9291
www.wdrake.com

Price: $3.99 for 100 gloves at the time of this writing.

Simple™ soap and shampoo

Order online from **The Garden Pharmacy** at:
    www.garden.co.uk/acatalog - search for Simple products
or from **Boots** at:
    http://www.boots.com/en/Simple/

Stevia (white crystalline extract)

NOW Natural Foods *(for older-style stevia, get this from your
    health food store)*
www.nowfoods.com

Allergy Adapt Inc. *(for next-generation stevia with almost no
    licorice-like taste)*
www.foodallergyandglutenfreeweightloss.com/stevia.html

Tortilla maker, electric

Chef Pro Tortilla Maker, available in 8 inch or 10 inch sizes, at http://www.amazon.com/Chef-Inch-Tortilla-Maker-Bread/dp/B002 HFQWH6

I have not used this tortilla maker because my Vitantonio model still works, although it is no longer being made. The Chef Pro is what Dr. Ruth Gornet-Irwin has and uses for her shot time tortillas. Read about why I trust her recommendation on page 72.

White sweet potato, cassava*, malanga, true yam, water chestnut, * and other "exotic" flours, cereals, pastas and prepared foods

Special Foods
9207 Shotgun Court
Springfield, Virginia 22153
(703) 644-0991
www.specialfoods.com

Note about Special Foods: The Special Foods website is down at the time of this writing and they are not answering their phone. This happened a few years ago, and they did begin accepting orders by phone again after about six months. See pages 72-73 for more about how to bake without them while we wait to see if they will be back again. Also, rather than baking, consider adding fresh cassava root and white sweet potatoes to your critical-3-day diet. Recipes are on pages 29-31.

*Cassava flour may be purchased from Ottos Naturals. See page 77. Water chestnut starch may be purchased from Asian grocery stores.

Index

Recipes appear in standard type;
informational sections appear in italics.

Books to Help Low Dose Immunotherapy Patients with Their Special Diets

The Ultimate Food Allergy Cookbook and Survival Guide: How to Cook with Ease for Food Allergies and Recover Good Health gives you everything you need to survive and recover from food allergies. It contains medical information about the diagnosis of food allergies, health problems that can be caused by food allergies, and your options for treatment. The book includes a rotation diet that is free from common food allergens such as wheat, milk, eggs, corn, soy, yeast, beef, legumes, citrus fruits, potatoes, tomatoes, and more. Instructions are given on how to personalize the standard rotation diet. It contains 500 recipes that fit the diet. Extensive reference sections include a listing of commercially prepared foods for allergy diets and sources for special foods, services, and products.

ISBN 978-1-887624-08-4 . . . . $24.95

***Allergy Cooking With Ease* (Revised Edition)**. This classic all-purpose allergy cookbook was out of print and now is making a comeback in a revised edition. It includes all the old favorite recipes of the first edition plus many new recipes and new foods. It contains over 300 recipes for baked goods, main dishes, soups, salads, vegetables, ethnic dishes, desserts, and more. Informational sections of the book are also updated, including the extensive "Sources" section.

ISBN 978-1-887624-10-7 . . . .$19.95

Gluten-Free Without Rice introduces you to gluten-free grains and grain alternatives other than rice such as teff, millet, sorghum, amaranth, quinoa, buckwheat, tapioca, arrowroot, potato starch, and more. It gives you over 75 delicious recipes for muffins, crackers, bread, pancakes, waffles, granola, main and side dishes, cookies, and desserts. Cook easily for a gluten-free diet without relying on rice

ISBN 978-1-887624-15-2 . . . . $9.95

Easy Breadmaking for Special Diets contains over 200 recipes for allergy, heart healthy, low fat, low sodium, yeast-free, controlled carbohydrate, diabetic, celiac, and low calorie diets. It includes recipes for breads of all kinds (including sourdough made with a wheat and gluten-free freeze dried starter), bread and tortilla based main dishes, and desserts. Use your bread machine, food processor, mixer, or electric tortilla maker to make the bread YOU need quickly and easily.

Third Edition – ISBN 978-1-887624-20-6 . . . . $19.95
Original Edition bargain book – ISBN 1-887624-02-3 . . . . $9.95

Allergy and Celiac Diets With Ease: Money and Time Saving Solutions for Food Allergy and Gluten-Free Diets provides solutions to both the economic and time challenges you face with your diet. This book contains over 160 money-saving, quick and easy recipes for allergy and celiac diets. Over 140 of them are gluten-free. It includes extensive reference sections including "Sources" and "Special Diet Resources" sections to help you find the foods you need. A list of helpful books and websites (even an online celiac/special diet restaurant search database) is also included.

ISBN 978-1-887624-17-6. . . . .$19.95

The Low Dose Immunotherapy Handbook: Recipes and Lifestyle Tips for Patients on LDA and EPD Treatment gives 80 recipes for patients on low dose immunotherapy treatment for their food allergies. It also includes organizational information to help you get ready for your shots.

ISBN 978-1-887624-07-7 . . . . $9.95

How to Cope With Food Allergies When You're Short on Time is a booklet of time saving tips and recipes to help you stick to your allergy diet with the least amount of time and effort.

$5.95 or FREE with the order of two other books

Order Form

Ship to:

Name: _____

Street address: _____

City, State, ZIP code: _____

Phone number (for questions about order): _____

Item	Quantity	Price	Total
Allergy Cooking with Ease		$19.95	
The Ultimate Food Allergy Cookbook & Survival Guide		$24.95	
Easy Breadmaking for Special Diets – Original Edition Bargain Book Third Edition		$9.95 $19.95	
The Low Dose Immunotherapy Handbook*		$9.95	
Write in additional books here:			
How to Cope with Food Allergies When You're Short on Time*		$5.95 or **FREE**	
Order any TWO of the first four books above or on the previous pages and get *How to Cope* **FREE!**	Subtotal		
	Shipping: See page 90 for chart		
	Colorado residents add 4.1% sales tax		
	Total		

Shipping:

    IF YOU ARE ORDERING JUST ONE BOOK, FOR SHIPPING ADD:

        $5.00 for any one of the first four (large, non-starred) books
           or other larger books described on the previous pages
        $3.00 for either of the last two (small, starred*) books

    TO ORDER MORE THAN ONE BOOK, FOR SHIPPING ADD:

        $7.00 for up to three non-starred (large) and two starred* books
        $9.00 for up to five non-starred and up to two starred* books

Call 303-666-8253 if you have questions about shipping calculations or large quantity orders.

Mail this order form and your check to:

Allergy Adapt, Inc.
1877 Polk Avenue
Louisville, CO 80027

**For more information about food allergies
or these and other books visit:**

www.food-allergy.org or

www.foodallergyandglutenfreeweightloss.com

For online orders, visit:

barnesandnoble.com or

amazon.com

www.ingramcontent.com/pod-product-compliance
Lightning Source LLC
Chambersburg PA
CBHW070903280326
41934CB00008B/1561